Medical Writing and Research Methodology for the Orthopaedic Surgeon

Cyril Mauffrey • Marius M. Scarlat

Editors

Medical Writing and Research Methodology for the Orthopaedic Surgeon

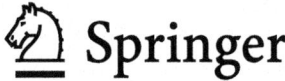

Springer

Editors
Cyril Mauffrey
Associate Director of Service
Director of Orthopaedic Trauma and Research
Denver Health Medical Center
Denver, Colorado
USA

Marius M. Scarlat
Departement Chirurgie Orthopédique
Clinique Chirurgicale St Michel
Toulon, France

ISBN 978-3-319-69349-1   ISBN 978-3-319-69350-7   (eBook)
https://doi.org/10.1007/978-3-319-69350-7

Library of Congress Control Number: 2017963007

Printed on acid-free paper

This Springer imprint is published by Springer Nature
The registered company is Springer International Publishing AG
The registered company address is: Gewerbestrasse 11, 6330 Cham, Switzerland

Foreword

The advancement of clinical care in orthopaedic surgery depends on high-quality clinical research transmitted to the practitioner community through clear medical writing. Drs. Mauffrey and Scarlat have assembled a highly experienced group of authors to address these issues. The author panel hails from the editorial board of major journals in the orthopaedic specialty including *Clinical Orthopaedics and Related Research, Injury, International Orthopaedics, The Journal of Bone and Joint Surgery*, and *the European Journal of Orthopaedic Surgery and Traumatology*. The chapters are succinctly outlined and address all the critical issues in both clear medical writing communication style and research design. Throughout the text of the chapters, there are multiple references made to the important tools for clinical research including CONSORT for randomized trials, STROBE for cohort studies, and PRISMA for systematic reviews and meta-analyses. The chapter on non-primary English speaking authors is of great value. Most medical publishing houses affiliated with these orthopaedic journals have services available to translate and edit manuscripts from non-English speakers, which are valuable tools at reasonable costs. Although one might think that the young practitioner beginning her or his research career would not be interested in matters of publication indices, the chapter on impact factor and Altmetrics is and will become increasingly so an important factor in the world of scholarly publication. The book provides much in the way of useful advice for the beginning clinical researcher, and I recommend it to all registrars and residents, young faculty beginning their clinical research careers, and experienced clinicians who are embarking on sharing their clinical experience with a broader audience of the orthopaedic community. I am sure that this publication will find broad acceptance in the orthopaedic community as we are critically dependent on improving our clinical research and communicating it effectively for now and in the future.

Marc F. Swiontkowski, MD
Professor, Department of Orthopaedic Surgery, University of Minnesota,
Editor-in-Chief, Journal of Bone and Joint Surgery,
Minneapolis, MN, USA

Contents

Contributors

Matthew P. Abdel Department of Orthopedic Surgery, Mayo Clinic, Rochester, MN, USA

Stuart A. Aitken Department of Orthopaedic Trauma, Foothills Medical Centre, Calgary, AB, Canada

Charles M. Court-Brown Department of Orthopaedic Trauma, University of Edinburgh, Edinburgh, UK

Peter V. Giannoudis Academic Department Trauma and Orthopaedic Surgery, School of Medicine, University of Leeds, Leeds, UK

Seth S. Leopold Clinical Orthopaedics and Related Research, University of Washington, Seattle, WA, USA

Cyril Mauffrey Department of Orthopaedics, Denver Health Medical Center, Denver, CO, USA

Andreas F. Mavrogenis First Department of Orthopaedics, Athens University Medical School, Athens, Greece

Matthieu Ollivier Department of Orthopedic Surgery, Mayo Clinic College of Medicine, Rochester, MN, USA

Georgios N. Panagopoulos First Department of Orthopaedics, Athens University Medical School, Athens, Greece

Costas Papakostidis Academic Department Trauma and Orthopaedic Surgery, School of Medicine, University of Leeds, Leeds, UK

Hans-Christoph Pape Department of Trauma, University of Zurich, Zurich, Switzerland

Fredric M. Pieracci Denver Health Medical Center, University of Colorado School of Medicine, Denver, CO, USA

Luca Pierannunzii Gaetano Pini Orthopaedic Institute, Milan, Italy

Andrew Quaile The Hampshire Clinic, Basingstoke, Hampshire, UK

Adam Sassoon Department of Orthopaedics and Sports Medicine, University of Washington, Seattle, WA, USA

Marius M. Scarlat Clinique St. Michel, Toulon, France

Philip F. Stahel Department of Orthopaedics, School of Medicine and Denver Health Medical Center, University of Colorado, Denver, CO, USA

Department of Neurosurgery, School of Medicine and Denver Health Medical Center, University of Colorado, Denver, CO, USA

Ryan Stancil Department of Orthopaedics and Sports Medicine, University of Washington, Seattle, WA, USA

Simon Tiziani Department of Trauma, University of Zurich, Zurich, Switzerland

Todd VanderHeiden Department of Orthopaedics, School of Medicine and Denver Health Medical Center, University of Colorado, Denver, CO, USA

Fraud in Publishing

Andreas F. Mavrogenis, Georgios N. Panagopoulos,
Cyril Mauffrey, and Marius M. Scarlat

1.1 Introduction

Since the first scientific journal appeared back in 1665 [1], medical publishing has gone a long way. Strict selection criteria, peer-reviewing, anti-fraud software, and pre-requisites for statistical validation of scientific work have all contributed to the steady production of an unparalleled number of high-quality manuscripts. No one debates the contribution that medical publishing has to the actual progress of science. As Drummond Rennie once wrote in one of the most prestigious medical journals *"… science does not exist until it is published…"* [2]. However, scientific misconduct or fraud represents an important issue in publishing. As Medicine remains essentially a career-driven discipline, institutional support and research funding largely depend on good reputation and prolificacy. As pressure for publishing becomes higher and higher and more emphasis is given to quantity rather than quality, researchers who are stressed to deliver tend to look for shortcuts. Despite the existence of austere ethical standards, reports of fraud have increased sharply in the last few decades. Unfortunately, most researchers believe that this is due to increased vigilance compared to the past [3].

There are many definitions of scientific misconduct (fraud) in medical writing and publishing [4]. The Royal College of Physicians of Edinburg defines scientific misconduct as *"…the behavior by a researcher, intentional or not, that falls short of good ethical and scientific standard…"* [5]. The UK Committee on Public Ethics (COPE) describes scientific misconduct as *"…the intention to cause others to*

A.F. Mavrogenis (✉) • G.N. Panagopoulos
First Department of Orthopaedics, National and Kapodistrian University of Athens,
School of Medicine, Athens, Greece
e-mail: afm@otenet.gr

C. Mauffrey
Department of Orthopaedics, Denver Health Medical Center, Denver, CO, USA

M.M. Scarlat
Clinique St. Michel, Toulon, France

© Springer International Publishing AG 2018
C. Mauffrey, M.M. Scarlat (eds.), *Medical Writing and Research Methodology for the Orthopaedic Surgeon*, https://doi.org/10.1007/978-3-319-69350-7_1

regard as true that which is not true…" [6]. The US Office of Research Integrity (ORI) reports that *"…research misconduct means fabrication, falsification, or plagiarism in proposing, performing, or reviewing research, or in reporting research results…"* (the FFP model) [7]. From a legal point of view, Protti et al. state that *"… scientific fraud is a deliberate misrepresentation by someone who knows the truth…"* [8].

Bad or fake research may misdirect the research of others. Therefore, scientific misconduct is not an issue to take lightly, as it might have serious consequences not only to the involved perpetrator or whistle-blower but also potentially devastating public health implications.

1.2   Types of Fraud in Publishing

In general, scientific misconduct in publishing includes three broad categories: fabrication, falsification, and plagiarism (the FFP model). However, this can only be seen as an oversimplification of the fraud that can take place in the field of publishing. As expected, many shades of gray exist, with the authors "con artists" having many tricks under their hat.

1.2.1   Fabrication

Fabrication is the most common form of fraud in medical research. It refers to the report of results that are completely made up. It literally involves the total or subtotal invention of data or information. This phenomenon is sometimes referred to as forging or dry-labbing [9], which does not only include made-up data but also the description of experiments that were never performed in the first place [10]. A minor form of fabrication is the use of fake or unrelated references, to give an argument a fake sense of widespread acceptance. A striking case of fabrication in publishing is the Pearce affair of a successfully reimplanted ectopic pregnancy that proved to be a complete figment of imagination [11].

1.2.2   Falsification

Falsification refers to manipulation and willfully distortion of research materials, methods or equipment, and/or alteration or omission of data or results such that the actual research is nothing but accurately reported. "Cooking" is a falsification fraud type that refers to retaining and analyzing selectively only the results that strengthen the research hypothesis under investigation while ignoring data that might weaken or disprove the results favored [10]. The later phenomenon is sometimes referred to as "suppression." "Trimming" is another falsification fraud that refers to smoothing any data irregularity that would make the research results less convincing or less pertinent for publication [10]. The case of the German nanotechnology scientist Jan

Hendrik Schön who authored more than 90 papers between 1998 and 2002, including 15 papers in Science and Nature, is probably one of the most representative examples of falsification [12–16].

Fabrication and falsification are often combined to produce a highly visible research. A major case of combined fabrication and falsification fraud in medical literature was the Wakefield affair, known as the MMR vaccine controversy [17–19]. The suggested relation of the MMR vaccine with Crohn's disease [17] and autism [18] proved numerous misgivings on the researcher's behalf; the original paper was retracted, and the author was struck off the UK medical register [19].

1.2.3   Plagiarism

The term plagiarism derives from the Latin word *plagium* meaning kidnapping a man [20]. The US Office of Research Integrity (ORI) defines plagiarism as *"…both the theft or misappropriation of intellectual property and the substantial unattributed textual copying of another's work…"* [21]. In this definition, the term substantial unattributed textual copying refers to the verbatim or nearly verbatim copying of sentences and paragraphs, which materially mislead the ordinary reader regarding the contributions of the author [21]. The World Association of Medical Editors (WAME) defines plagiarism as *"…copying six consecutive words in a continuous set of 30 used characters…"* [20, 22]. In simple terms, plagiarism refers to the classic practice of "copy and paste"; it is synonymous with appropriation of the ideas, methods, results, or plain words of others without giving appropriate credit. Therefore, to avoid plagiarism, the use or report of another researcher's work or words should be adequately referenced; any quotation reported ad verbatim should be in quotation marks if six or more consecutive words are used. Failing to do those two simple tasks makes a document very likely to be red flagged as being a product of plagiarism.

Masic published a list of ten different types of plagiarism and how to prevent it. These include "cloning" (submitting someone else's work, fully transcribed), "ctrl-c" (copying without alterations text from a single source), "find-replace" (only changing key words or phrases), "remix" (paraphrasing or combining phrases from multiple sources), "recycle" (reusing one's own work), "hybrid" (combing perfectly cited sources with the copied without citation), "mash-up" (blending copied material from multiple sources), "error 404" (quoting fictional or inaccurate sources), "aggregator" (proper citation but lack of any original work), and "retweet" (proper citation but too much text from the original) [22]. Citation plagiarism refers to failure to appropriately credit prior discoverers, so as to give an improper sense of priority [23]. It is also referred to as "citation amnesia," "disregard syndrome," "bibliographic negligence" [23], and the Matthew effect or Stigler's law [24, 25]. A dear consequence of this can be the inadvertent reassignment of credit from the original discoverer to a better-known researcher [24, 25]. Probably the most representative example of plagiarism is the case of an Iraqi medical researcher who copied entire articles that had already been published, modified the title, replaced the authors' names with his own, and submitted the manuscripts to less well-known journals. In this way, he succeeded in accumulating publications and joining scientific societies and prestigious institutions until his lack of knowledge was exposed [26–29].

1.3   Authorship Issues

Another form of scientific misconduct involves maneuvering the authorship. This type of fraud includes many different practices such as "guest authorship," "gift authorship," "ghost authorship," "coercion authorship," and others [30–37]. Guest authorship refers to using the name of a well-known researcher in an effort to change the status accorded to the article and increase the chances of publication. A striking example of guest authorship is the Darsee affair in the 1980s; 55 of his ultimately retracted articles carried the name of his famous mentor who had little knowledge of their content [30–33]. Gift authorship is governed by the principle of reciprocity; authorship is offered as a gift in view of a future counter-gift, to encourage future collaborations, maintain good relations, or return a favor [34–36]. Ghost authorship or ghostwriting is the fact when someone else other than the named authors makes a major contribution; typically, this is done to mask contribution from drug companies, so as to hide a potential conflict of interest [35, 36]. Coercion authorship occurs when "superiors" with no direct involvement in a given research demand to or presume that they should be authors of any article originating within their department [36, 37]. A similar occurrence is inappropriate allocation of credit, where author rank does not correspond to the relative weight of individual author contributions.

1.4   Image Manipulation

The widespread use of photo editing software has given birth to yet another form of scientific misconduct, namely, image manipulation. This type of fraud may include splicing together different image to represent a single experiment, partially changing brightness or contrast, concealing information included in an image, or showing only a part of the image to cover any unwanted portion [38–42]. One Nature paper published in 2009 was reported to contain almost 20 separate instances of image fraud from a molecular experiment [43]. An anonymous internet user created a blog and uploaded a YouTube® video that demonstrated more than 60 manipulated images from 24 papers published from the lab in question [43, 44].

1.5   Collateral Practices

Redundant publication occurs when two or more papers, without cross-reference, share the same hypothesis, data, discussion points, or conclusions. Although previous publication of an abstract during the proceedings of meetings does not preclude subsequent submission for publication, full disclosure should be made at the time of submission. Types of redundant fraud are "salami" publishing, "templating," "shot-gunning," and "self-citation."

Salami publishing is a well-known practice of scientific misconduct. It consists of dividing the results of a research project into a series of articles (least publishable units) in order to maximize the number of potential publications [45–47]. This practice is considered to the least questionable [48–52].

Templating is considered a unique form of plagiarism that refers to copying not the ideas, methods, or science of others but essentially using the same format, structure, or similar phrasing. This method is usually followed by inexperienced, non-English-speaking authors, who tend to adapt their own submissions to the optimal structure of articles of others [45, 46].

Shotgunning refers to the simultaneous submission of the same research article to multiple journals [45]. This leads to the occurrence of duplicate or redundant publication, which is still considered misconduct, under what is known as the Ingelfinger rule [53–55].

Self-citation is defined in the *Journal Citation Report (JCR)* as referring to articles from the same journal or the same author. While this phenomenon might be acceptable if done occasionally, it can also be overused to increase the status and academic performance of an individual researcher [1, 56]. Additionally, excessive self-citation can indicate a manipulation by editors to increase the IF of their own journal [1]. One journal's IF was boosted 18 ranks by one paper containing 303 self-citations. Both journals involved were given a severe warning, and the next IFs published in June 2007 showed a decrease in their ranking [57]. Manipulating the IF can have serious consequences, such as affecting decisions on where to publish and who to promote or hire; awarding of research funding, grants, scholarships, and fellowships; allocating salary bonuses; or evaluating postgraduate courses by bureaucrats that usually ask for a simple metric to determine their decision-making process [58–60]. There are many ways a journal can skew the IF to its favor. Falagas et al. published an article in 2008, presenting a list of ten editorial policies that can achieve just that, including coercing self-citation, favoring review articles, rejecting negative or confirmatory studies, and publishing "hot" topics, among others [56]. A striking example is given by the specialist journal *Folia Phoniatrica et Logopedica*. This journal published an editorial in 2007 citing all its articles from 2005 to 2006, intended as a protest against the IF game. This editorial increased the IF of the journal from 0.66 to 1.44. However, rather than sending a message, the journal was penalized, by not being included in the 2008–2009 JCR [61, 62].

1.6   Countermeasures Implementation

Even though, at a first glance, scientific misconduct feels overwhelming, it is true that the scientific community has already gone a long way with fraud prevention and detection. A robust peer-review process, put forward by most scientific journals, constitutes a first obstacle for potential perpetrators. Furthermore, regulatory bodies establishing guidelines have been instituted around the world. Since the establishment of ORI in the USA in 1992 and COPE in the UK in 1997, many National Bodies for Ethics in Science currently exist in all European and North American countries. Whistle-blowers are protected by clauses of confidentiality. Many journals now validate research results with a dedicated statistical analysis, so to avoid fabrication and falsification. Plagiarism and image manipulation can now easily be detected with appropriate software such as TurnitIn®, SafeAssign®, CrossCheck®, Déjà vu®, and eTBlast®.

Combating fraud in publishing is not only a matter of good and bad literature. Eventually, bad references will be cited and may drive scientific research toward a wrong direction. Therefore, in a scientific world of prolificacy-driven academic careers, it is essential that scientists focus on quality rather than quantity.

References

1. Mavrogenis AF, Ruggieri P, Papagelopoulos PJ. Self-citation in publishing. Clin Orthop Relat Res. 2010;468:2803–7. https://doi.org/10.1007/s11999-010-1480-8.
2. Rennie D. The present state of medical journals. Lancet. 1998;352(Suppl 2):SII18–22.
3. Van Noorden R. Science publishing: the trouble with retractions. Nature. 2011;478:26–8. https://doi.org/10.1038/478026a.
4. Nylenna M, Andersen D, Dahlquist G, Sarvas M, Aakvaag A. Handling of scientific dishonesty in the Nordic countries. National committees on scientific dishonesty in the Nordic countries. Lancet. 1999;354:57–61.
5. Evans S. How common is it? Joint consensus conference on misconduct. Biomed Res. 2000;30(Suppl. 7):1.
6. Promoting integrity in research publication. Norfolk: Committee on Publication Ethics, COPE. http://publicationethics.org. Accessed 10 Sept 2015.
7. Office of Research Integrity. Definition of research misconduct. http://ori.hhs.gov/definition-misconduct. Accessed 10 Sept 2015.
8. Protti M. Policing fraud and deceit: the legal aspects of misconduct in scientific inquiry. J Infor Ethics. 1996;5:59–71.
9. Shapiro MF. Data audit by a regulatory agency: its effect and implication for others. Account Res. 1992;2:219–29. https://doi.org/10.1080/08989629208573818.
10. Jaffer U, Cameron AE. Deceit and fraud in medical research. Int J Surg. 2006;4:122–6. https://doi.org/10.1016/j.ijsu.2006.02.004.
11. Lock S. Lessons from the Pearce affair: handling scientific fraud. BMJ. 1995;310:1547–8.
12. Brumfiel G. Misconduct finding at bell labs shakes physics community. Nature. 2002;419:419–21. https://doi.org/10.1038/419419a.
13. Brumfiel G. Bell labs launches inquiry into allegations of data duplication. Nature. 2002; 417:367–8. https://doi.org/10.1038/417367a.
14. Grant P. Is a bell tolling for bell labs? Nature. 2002;417:789. https://doi.org/10.1038/417789a.
15. Service RF. Scientific misconduct. Bell labs fires star physicist found guilty of forging data. Science. 2002;298:30–1. https://doi.org/10.1126/science.298.5591.30.
16. Service RF. Bell labs. Winning streak brought awe, and then doubt. Science. 2002;297:34–7. https://doi.org/10.1126/science.297.5578.34.
17. Thompson NP, Montgomery SM, Pounder RE, Wakefield AJ. Is measles vaccination a risk factor for inflammatory bowel disease? Lancet. 1995;345:1071–4.
18. Wakefield AJ, Murch SH, Anthony A, Linnell J, Casson DM, Malik M, Berelowitz M, Dhillon AP, Thomson MA, Harvey P, Valentine A, Davies SE, Walker-Smith JA. Ileal-lymphoid-nodular hyperplasia, non-specific colitis, and pervasive developmental disorder in children. Lancet. 1998;351:637–41.

19. Godlee F, Smith J, Marcovitch H. Wakefield's article linking MMR vaccine and autism was fraudulent. BMJ. 2011;342:c7452. https://doi.org/10.1136/bmj.c7452.
20. Masic I. Plagiarism in scientific publishing. Acta Inform Med. 2012;20:208–13. https://doi.org/10.5455/aim.2012.20.208-213.
21. ORI policy on plagiarism. https://ori.hhs.gov/ori-policy-plagiarism. Accessed 10 Sept 2015.
22. Masic I. Plagiarism in scientific research and publications and how to prevent it. Mater Soc. 2014;26:141–6. https://doi.org/10.5455/msm.2014.26.141-146.
23. Garfield E (2002) Demand citation vigilance. http://www.garfield.library.upenn.edu/papers/demandcitationvigilance012102.html. Accessed 12 Sept 2015.
24. Merton RK. The Matthew effect in science: the reward and communication systems of science are considered. Science. 1968;159:56–63. https://doi.org/10.1126/science.159.3810.56.
25. Kern SE. Whose hypothesis? Ciphering, sectorials, D lesions, freckles and the operation of Stigler's law. Cancer Biol Ther. 2002;1:571–81.
26. Alsabti EAK. Massachusetts v. Alsabti. Science. 1989;245:1046. https://doi.org/10.1126/science.1046-c.
27. Broad WJ. Charges of piracy follow alsabti. Science. 1980;210:291. https://doi.org/10.1126/science.210.4467.291.
28. Broad W, Wade N. Betrayers of the truth. In: Touchstone book. New York: Simon and Schuster; 1983.
29. Miller DJ, Hersen M. Research fraud in the behavioral and biomedical sciences. New York, N.Y: Wiley; 1992.
30. Bonnet F, Samama CM. Cases of fraud in publications: from Darsee to Poldermans. Presse Med. 2012;41:816–20. https://doi.org/10.1016/j.lpm.2012.04.019.
31. Kochan CA, Budd JM. The persistence of fraud in the literature: the Darsee case. J Am Soc Inf Sci. 1992;43:488–93. https://doi.org/10.1002/(SICI)1097-4571(199208)43:7<488::AID-ASI3>3.0.CO;2-7.
32. Relman AS. Lessons from the Darsee affair. N Engl J Med. 1983;308:1415–7. https://doi.org/10.1056/NEJM198306093082311.
33. Tynan M, Anderson RH. Different lessons from the Darsee affair? Int J Cardiol. 1984;5:9–11.
34. Pontille D, Torny D. Behind the scenes of scientific articles: defining categories of fraud and regulating cases. Rev Epidemiol Sante Publique. 2012;60:247–53. https://doi.org/10.1016/j.respe.2012.06.395.
35. Kempers RD. Ethical issues in biomedical publications. Fertil Steril. 2002;77:883–8.
36. Claxton LD. Scientific authorship. Part 2. History, recurring issues, practices, and guidelines. Mutat Res. 2005;589:31–45. https://doi.org/10.1016/j.mrrev.2004.07.002.
37. Claxton LD. Scientific authorship. Part 1. A window into scientific fraud? Mutat Res. 2005;589:17–30. https://doi.org/10.1016/j.mrrev.2004.07.003.
38. Parrish D, Noonan B. Image manipulation as research misconduct. Sci Eng Ethics. 2009;15:161–7. https://doi.org/10.1007/s11948-008-9108-z.
39. Martin C, Blatt M. Manipulation and misconduct in the handling of image data. Plant Cell. 2013;25:3147–8. https://doi.org/10.1105/tpc.113.250980.
40. Hollyfield JG. Manuscript fabrication, image manipulation and plagiarism. Exp Eye Res. 2012;94:1–2. https://doi.org/10.1016/j.exer.2011.10.009.
41. Couzin-Frankel J. Image manipulation. Author of popular blog that charged fraud unmasked. Science. 2013;339:132. https://doi.org/10.1126/science.339.6116.132.
42. Astaneh B, Masoumi S. Image manipulation; how far is too far. J Pak Med Assoc. 2013;63:929–30.
43. Katolab image-fraud. http://katolab-imagefraud.blogspot.co.uk/2012/01/dna-demethylation-in-hormone-induced.html. Accessed 12 Sept 2015.
44. Alleged image fraud by Shigeaki Kato lab at the University of Tokyo (Alleged research misconduct). http://www.youtube.com/watch?v=FXaOqwanWnU. Accessed 13 Sept 2015.
45. Rogers LF. Salami slicing, shotgunning, and the ethics of authorship. Am J Roentgenol. 1999;173:265. https://doi.org/10.2214/ajr.173.2.10430115.
46. Gilbert FJ, Denison AR. Research misconduct. Clin Radiol. 2003;58:499–504.

47. Broad WJ. The publishing game: getting more for less. Science. 1981;211:1137–9.
48. Jackson D, Walter G, Daly J, Cleary M. Editorial: multiple outputs from single studies: acceptable division of findings vs. 'salami' slicing. J Clin Nurs. 2014;23(1–2). https://doi.org/10.1111/jocn.12439.
49. Klein AA, Pozniak A, Pandit JJ. Salami slicing or living off the fat? Justifying multiple publications from a single HIV dataset. Anaesthesia. 2014;69:195–8. https://doi.org/10.1111/anae.12603.
50. Norman G. Data dredging, salami-slicing, and other successful strategies to ensure rejection: twelve tips on how to not get your paper published. Adv Health Sci Educ Theory Pract. 2014;19:1–5. https://doi.org/10.1007/s10459-014-9494-8.
51. Pierson CA. Salami slicing--how thin is the slice? J Am Assoc Nurse Pract. 2015;27:65. https://doi.org/10.1002/2327-6924.12210.
52. Supak Smolcic V. Salami publication: definitions and examples. Biochem Med. 2013;23:237–41.
53. Netland PA. Ethical authorship and the Ingelfinger rule in the digital age. Ophthalmology. 2013;120:1111–2. https://doi.org/10.1016/j.ophtha.2013.02.013.
54. Harnad S. Ingelfinger over-ruled. Lancet. 2000;356:s16.
55. Germenis AE. Beyond the Ingelfinger rule: the intellectual property ethics after the end of biomedical journals' monopoly. Med Inform Internet Med. 1999;24:165–70.
56. Falagas ME, Alexiou VG. The top-ten in journal impact factor manipulation. Arch Immunol Ther Exp. 2008;56:223–6. https://doi.org/10.1007/s00005-008-0024-5.
57. Kirchhof B, Bornfeld N, Grehn F. The delicate topic of the impact factor Graefe's. Arch Clin Exp Ophthalmol. 2007;245:925–7.
58. Cash-per-publication. Nature. 2006;441:786. https://doi.org/10.1038/441786a.
59. PLoS Medicine Editors. The impact factor game. It is time to find a better way to assess the scientific literature. PLoS Med. 2006;3:e291. https://doi.org/10.1371/journal.pmed.0030291.
60. Whitehouse GH. Impact factors: facts and myths. Eur Radiol. 2002;12:715–7. https://doi.org/10.1007/s00330-001-1212-2.
61. Schutte HK, Svec JG. Reaction of folia Phoniatrica et Logopaedica on the current trend of impact factor measures. Folia Phoniatr Logop. 2007;59:281–5. https://doi.org/10.1159/000108334.
62. Foo JY. Impact of excessive journal self-citations: a case study on the folia Phoniatrica et Logopaedica journal. Sci Eng Ethics. 2011;17:65–73. https://doi.org/10.1007/s11948-009-9177-7.

The Use of English and Its Editing

2

Andrew Quaile

2.1 Introduction

I act as Content Editor for International Orthopaedics which is written in English and what I would consider as the original language. English is also the language used in the majority of prestigious Orthopaedic Journals. This is a historical fact and not one for discussion in the chapter. English by its very nature is a mixture of languages with influences from Latin, Anglo-Saxon, Norse and most recently French. It has been said that 60% of English has French roots, and it has been further influenced by the American adaptions. Journals can therefore vary with the 'English' they use. American Journals will tend to use the American version and British Journals the British. Despite vigorous debate the English actually used is secondary to the purpose of 'getting the message across'. This chapter attempts to dispel the myths of that debate and empower authors to provide an entertaining, educational and publishable article.

2.2 What Are the Challenges?

The challenges facing authors, in order to get an article published in a prestigious Orthopaedic Journal, are manifold. It should be obvious that a well-presented article has a much better chance of being published and cited. A shambolic and poorly written article has a lower chance of being accepted even if the science is good. That is because the message has to be understood by the readership of the journal and therefore needs a consistent recognisable style. It does not need to have the prose of Shakespeare, but it does need to be readable and furthermore entertaining enough to keep the reader's attention. This should be automatic, but in my experience of both

A. Quaile
The Hampshire Clinic, Basingstoke, Hampshire, UK
e-mail: andrew@spine-works.com

© Springer International Publishing AG 2018
C. Mauffrey, M.M. Scarlat (eds.), *Medical Writing and Research Methodology for the Orthopaedic Surgeon*, https://doi.org/10.1007/978-3-319-69350-7_2

reviewing orthopaedic articles and content editing, there are many poorly written articles, some of which need a virtual rewrite to make enough sense to be published. Such interference runs the risk of changing the sense of the article which is clearly something that should be avoided. The way language is used is a major part of getting your message across to colleagues. Your article should, therefore, adopt the same techniques used in all walks of life, business and politics. You are trying to persuade the journal editor, reviewer and eventually readership of its value to you and to them. A well-written and well-organised article is far more likely to do so.

If English, in all its forms, is not your native tongue, it would be an advantage to have a native English speaker review your article. If there is no one immediately available, there is online support available from a number of firms who can supply translation services, and indeed some journals offer a similar type of service. There are also services such as 'Google' translate. Care needs to be exercised here as the standard of translation is actually not very good, and it will tend to default to the American version of English which would need changing to the British version if the article is offered to a British journal or indeed International Orthopaedics. Articles written in Word tend to autocorrect to the American version of English unless you are able to change the parameters of the programme. It should also be recognised that Orthopaedic Journals are distributed throughout the world and to colleagues whose English is minimal or at least not advanced. The language used therefore has to be able to get the concepts in the article across in a simple and straightforward fashion. One British journal describes informing 'the man from Mandalay' as a way of getting authors to understand their audience. Journals are not just read in New York and London. There must therefore be a responsibility to educate the reader in the English language by ensuring what is written is indeed 'good English'.

2.3   Tips and Tricks for a Successful Submission

Consistency, consistency and consistency would be the first and foremost piece of advice here. It is remarkable the number of articles I see during content editing that use different spelling or different punctuation for the same word in the same paragraph. The article should be one which educates and is relevant to the readership. It can only do so if the message contained is clearly communicated and understood.

It should be recognised that there are two main forms of English, and therefore some research needs to be carried out prior to submission to understand the style of the target journal. This style can be understood by both reading the journal and by reading the instructions to authors which all journals publish. It is remarkable how rarely this is done. Obviously as orthopaedic surgeons, we want to concentrate on the science, but much pain will be reduced if the instructions are read. Some example of the different spelling used would be orthopaedic/orthopedic, paediatric/pediatric, tumour/tumor, fibre/fiber, oedema/ edema and aetiology/etiology. The British version is the first example. The use of 'ise' at the end words rather than 'ize' is another British form of English. Whilst it would not be regarded as a critical problem if the article was presented in the American form of English to a British journal, it would tend to show that the style of the journal had not been appreciated.

The title of the article is very important as it is both the selling point of the article and the way it is identified via search engines such as Pubmed and Google Scholar. The title will also have relevance to the journal's impact factor and the number of citations received. It therefore needs to accurately describe the contents and be relevant to the paper. It should be relatively short and punchy whilst delivering the necessary description. Think of a newspaper headline. There should be no abbreviations, no numerals or no acronyms, and furthermore dates should be fully written out. As much thought should go into the title as the rest of the paper as this is its selling point.

Phrases should be carefully constructed and the use of language skilful. Phrases such as 'this present paper' should more properly be 'this paper/our paper'. The word 'surgeries' does not exist in British English as the plural of surgery. It should more properly be operations, operative procedures or indeed surgery. Similarly operated becomes operated upon or perhaps treated.

Hyphens and their use is the greatest problem I come across in performing content editing. They are very poorly understood and used inconsistently. There is a distressing tendency to invent words in orthopaedics by joining them together, arriving at a mega-word which is impossible to say or indeed understand. The purpose of hyphens is to aid understanding, not to make comprehension more difficult. They are supposed to be used in compound words to show the components have a consistent meaning such as mother-in-law. They are most commonly used in orthopaedics to join a prefix such as intra-operative, post-operative, pre-operative and post-traumatic. Not using a hyphen in these situations produces an ugly word and also places two vowels together in some situations, which should be avoided wherever possible. Hyphens are further used as word breaks in editing. The use of hyphens should be consistent, aiding understanding and comprehension of your article. Sadly, this is not often the case.

Numbers should be written out from one to ten, apart from when in brackets, and from 11 onwards in numeral form. This largely relates to numbers used with periods of time, numbers of patients, implants and so on. Numbers used with weights and measures, percentages and fractions tend to be expressed as numerals.

Furthermore, it is better to express time in words as it seems illogical to write out years, months, days and hours but not to write out minutes and seconds. It also aids understanding as, for instance, the abbreviation 'min.' could mean minimum. Weights and measures have their own well-developed abbreviations.

2.4 Common Mistakes and How to Prevent Them

The most common mistake by far is lack of consistency of spelling or language throughout an article. That shows lack of editing by the author and therefore lack of care in its production. It also reveals a 'slap-dash' tendency which devalues the article and makes the reader wonder about the underlying science and care taken in the research it purports to represent. It is therefore vital to proof-read your article before submission. Errors of language can be corrected during the content editing process, but lack of consistency in the use of spelling, punctuation or language conveys a careless attitude and should be avoided at all costs. Such lack of attention to detail could be terminal for your paper.

Time spent reviewing your title and comparing it with other articles on the same subject will help in having your article published and recognised by search engines. Other similar articles are likely to have been quoted with your references which will act as an 'aide memoire'.

Having your article reviewed to check the language and content either by a native English speaker or by an English-speaking colleague will help iron out obvious deficiencies and to produce a well-honed article which stands more chance of publication.

2.5   Take-Home Message

1. Clarity of language is crucial to get your message across.
2. Have your manuscript read by native English speakers.
3. Reviewers will tend to reject a paper if it is not well written.
4. Spelling and grammar mistakes reduce the impact of your paper.
5. Understand and follow 'instructions to authors' from the relevant journal.

Developing a Sound Research Methodology

3

Luca Pierannunzii

3.1 Introduction

A sound methodology is essential to produce publishable results. Both original articles and systematic reviews are research-based manuscripts. In this chapter we will focus on the preparation of a clinical study, which is reported through an original article, while we will ignore Systematic Reviews methodology, since it will be dealt with in a subsequent chapter ("systematic reviews and meta-analyses").

The main quality of biomedical research is the originality of the subject: this means that studies should answer novel, important research questions [1]. Finding original research questions represents the true challenge for most scholars, as "original" in medical literature is the combination of three features: "unpublished," "not derivable from previous publications," and "topical and clinically relevant."

The clinical relevance is the condition next to novelty: orthopedic research is mostly clinical or preclinical, which implies that some manuscripts, although truly novel, may be rejected by editors of clinical journals simply because the results cannot be translated into tangible consequences for the clinical practice (Fig. 3.1).

The PICO method [2] is helpful in developing adequate research questions, as in this example:

P	Population/patient	Patients over 40 with hip osteoarthritis Tönnis grade 2–3 and femoroacetabular impingement
I	Intervention/indicator	Hip arthroscopy
C	Comparator/control	Total hip arthroplasty (THA)
O	Outcome	Patient's satisfaction (NRS) and mHHS

Question: Do patients over 40 with hip osteoarthritis Tönnis 2–3 and femoroacetabular impingement after hip arthroscopy have subjective and clinic-functional benefits non-inferior to THA?

L. Pierannunzii
Gaetano Pini Orthopaedic Institute, Milan, Italy
e-mail: LMCPierannunzii@hotmail.com

© Springer International Publishing AG 2018
C. Mauffrey, M.M. Scarlat (eds.), *Medical Writing and Research Methodology for the Orthopaedic Surgeon*, https://doi.org/10.1007/978-3-319-69350-7_3

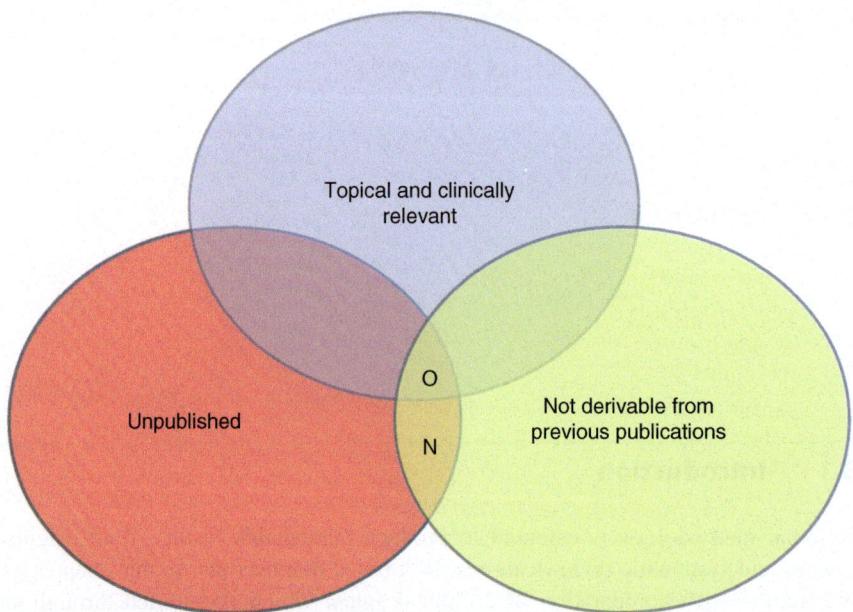

Fig. 3.1 Diagram showing the relationship between original (O), novel (N) and "unpublished," "not derivable from previous publications," and "topical and clinically relevant"

The clinical studies are commonly classified in *experimental* and *observational* [3]: the former exposes the subjects to a factor that potentially modifies their health status (a surgical procedure, a pharmacological treatment, a rehab protocol); the latter observes the results of an exposure that has already occurred independently of the research (e.g., having received a certain type of joint replacement, suffering from a disease like osteoporosis or osteoarthritis, smoking, etc.).

Experimental studies are always prospective and possibly comparative: if the allocation is randomized, the study is a RCT (randomized controlled trial). Sometimes ethical concerns or low budget keep researchers from choosing a RCT, that otherwise would guarantee the highest level of evidence.

Observational studies are further divided into cohort (i.e., prospectively or retrospectively followed from the exposure to the outcome), case-control (i.e., retrospectively investigated from the outcome to the exposure), and cross-sectional study (where outcome and exposure are detected simultaneously).

Specific guidelines to report observational and experimental studies are, respectively, STROBE (STrengthening the Reporting of OBservational studies in Epidemiology [4]) and CONSORT (CONsolidated Standards Of Reporting Trials [5]).

3.2   What Are the Challenges?

- Assessing the originality and refining the research hypothesis requires a systematic search throughout the main biomedical databases (PubMed/

MEDLINE, Google, Web of Science, Scopus, etc.) to ascertain that the subject was not satisfactorily addressed by previous studies. (1) If many articles can be found describing well-designed studies and leading to consistent conclusions, probably the subject is not as original as we thought, and there is little need of further evidence. (2) If many articles show conflicting results, we should try to overcome possible errors and bias designing a study with higher level of evidence [6]. In case level 1 or 2 studies are already reported, probably the question might be better answered with a systematic review. (3) If the search results in a few studies with variable/uncertain conclusions, then the subject is insufficiently explored indeed and is likely to deserve a focused investigation.

- Designing a clinical study is challenging, and most orthopedic surgeons need the assistance of a biostatistician to plan the study properly. Methodological errors such as an undersized sample or a wrong test may compromise the reliability of conclusions. For this reason *the statistician should be consulted prior to collecting data* and not afterward.
- The knowledge of the existing literature is important to calculate the sample size and to decide how to measure the outcome: the more our data is homogeneous with other Authors', the easier it will be to compare results and produce meta-analyses. Data collection should be careful, especially if it involves a degree of manual skills or discernment. In these cases outcome-related measures should possibly be repeated by two examiners, and both intra-rater and inter-rater agreements should be calculated. Blindness or even double-blindness is recommended when ethically applicable.
- Authors are encouraged to register their protocols as soon as possible, anyway before subjects' enrollment, through www.clinicaltrial.gov or other registries listed in the International Clinical Trials Registry Platform (ICTRP) http://www.who.int/ictrp/network/primary/en/ [7]. This registration is compulsory whenever the study design is experimental and prospective.
- The ethical requirements for research on human subjects have to be timely fulfilled before the beginning of the study: in the manuscript the Authors are requested to state that their investigation complies with the Declaration of Helsinki [8], that all the participants signed an informed consent, and that the responsible Ethics Committee/Institutional Review Board approved the protocol. Not fulfilling just one of these three conditions might result in an editorial rejection on ethical ground, unless the exemption is guaranteed by law or other national regulations [9].

3.3   From a Clinical Study to an Original Article

Scientific articles should always be neat and concise, from the title through the abstract to the full text. Authors have to adhere to methods and data, presenting them in an orderly fashion through the IMRaD structure [10].

The *title* should not only be informative but also concise and engaging; the *abstract* is a short but complete summary, with mention of purpose, methodology, results, and conclusion: "writing a good abstract is not abstract writing" [11].

The *Introduction* should briefly summarize the background knowledge and justify why this study is needed (gap of knowledge) and why its results may be clinically relevant. At the end of the introduction, the Author should always state the hypothesis.

Materials and Methods is the section where the protocol of the study is described both from a clinical point of view (disease, treatment, follow-up) and from a statistical point of view (tests, alpha, power, sample size, etc.). Each outcome (endpoint) listed in *Materials and Methods* should correspond to data in *Results*. Check the ratio 1:1 between endpoints anticipated in *Materials and Methods* and data reported in *Results*. The *Results* section usually is the only one with no references.

The *Discussion* is the place where Authors summarize their results, compare them with results found in literature, explicit strengths and weaknesses of their work, and state the conclusions (in other words whether the hypothesis is verified or not).

In regard to the length of the manuscript, *as long as you need, but as short as you can* is the best recommendation. Verbosity diverts readers' attention and usually aims at masking lack of contents. Scientific writing is a technical writing where each sentence conveys a piece of information. An original article is not supposed to be read from the beginning to the end like a narrative paper; readers should be able to find quickly the information they need simply knowing where it should be located.

3.4 Common Mistakes and How to Prevent Them

Data presentation is critical and often defective or redundant. It should be statistically complete and formally compliant with Instructions for Authors: i.e., continuous variables will be expressed as mean value ± standard deviation and range or, in other journals, as mean value, 95% confidence interval and range. When possible and convenient, data will be summarized in tables, avoiding duplicating it in the text. Lastly, in *Results* it's better not to write next to statements "$p < 0.05$" because it is obvious if 0.05 is your level α; Authors should write instead the exact value of p (i.e., "$p = 0.026$").

Another common mistake is describing the samples (i.e., demographics and confounding factors) in *Results*, while they should be described in *Materials and Methods*. Even if a statistical analysis was necessary to ascertain that the group of patients was comparable to the group of controls, this information belongs to *Materials and Methods*.

Lastly, it ought to be reminded that fractionating a large study into minimum publishable units (or MPU) is a questionable research practice very close to the self-plagiarism and might lead to the rejection of the following manuscripts.

3.5   Take-Home Message

The scientific research methodology is a process that we learn both regularly reading scientific articles and participating in clinical research from the very beginning of our careers. These are the key points:

- Be curious: often researchers are driven to brilliant topics merely by curiosity.
- Scan regularly the up-to-date literature, to recognize emerging and/or controversial topics timely.
- Be familiar with biomedical databases and with search engines, to check the originality of the topic and find akin articles (that constitute the background knowledge).
- Ask the assistance of a statistician to elaborate the protocol. However it is recommended to be comfortable with basic statistics, at least to have a profitable relationship with the statistician.
- Fulfill the obligations (trial registration, ethical clearance).
- Find sufficient resources to guarantee the financial coverage of the study.
- Perform the study in a reasonable period of time, to preserve the topicality of the subject.
- Prepare an original article, to share the results with the scientific community. The use of templates (i.e., those made available by several journals together with Instructions for Authors) or checklists for proper reporting clinical studies [4, 5] will prevent you from dropping important pieces of information.

References

1. Richardson WS, Wilson MC, Nishikawa J, Hayward RS. The well-built clinical question: a key to evidence-based decisions. ACP J Club. 1995;123(3):A12–3.
2. Bragge P. Asking good clinical research questions and choosing the right study design. Injury. 2010;41(Suppl 1):S3–6.
3. Grimes DA, Schulz KF. An overview of clinical research: the lay of the land. Lancet. 2002;359:57–61.
4. STROBE (STrengthening the Reporting of OBservational studies in Epidemiology). http://www.strobe-statement.org. Accessed 20 Aug 2016.
5. CONSORT (CONsolidated Standards Of Reporting Trials). http://www.consort-statement.org/. Accessed 20 Aug 2016.
6. OCEBM Levels of Evidence Working Group. The Oxford 2011 Levels of Evidence. Oxford Centre for Evidence-Based Medicine. http://www.cebm.net/index.aspx?o=5653. Accessed 20 Aug 2016.
7. International Clinical Trials Registry Platform (ICTRP). http://www.who.int/ictrp/network/primary/en/. Accessed 20 Aug 2016.
8. World Medical Association (1964, amended in 2013) Declaration of Helsinki. http://www.wma.net/en/30publications/10policies/b3/. Accessed 20 Aug 2016.
9. Pierannunzii L. Ethical requirements for musculoskeletal research involving human subjects. J Orthop Traumatol. 2015;16(4):265–8.
10. International Steering Committee of Medical Editors. Uniform requirements for manuscripts submitted to biomedical journals. Br Med J. 1979;1:532–5.
11. Baue A. Writing a good abstract is not abstract writing. Arch Surg. 1979;114(1):11–2.

What Editors and Reviewers Look for: Tips for Successful Research Publication

4

Ryan Stancil, Seth S. Leopold, and Adam Sassoon

4.1 Introduction

Scientific reporting of original biomedical research can and should be demanding. After all, the health and well-being of our patients depends not just on the rigor of the studies being reported but also on our ability to understand who was included in those studies, how they were treated, and how endpoints were assessed. Clarity, therefore, is critical.

But demanding need not mean difficult. Sensible principles underlie the reporting standards that journals use and tools can make presenting the material much easier on authors. This chapter highlights the common challenges authors face as they set out to present their work for publication in peer-reviewed journals, offers some tips to help mitigate those challenges, identifies several common mistakes that recur in scientific reporting, and proposes some ways to avoid them.

4.2 What Are the Challenges?

Undoubtedly, the challenges vary—based on the authors' experiences as researchers, the resources available, the topics being studied, and countless other factors. But we

R. Stancil (✉) • A. Sassoon
Department of Orthopaedics and Sports Medicine,
University of Washington, Seattle, WA, USA
e-mail: ryands@uw.edu

S.S. Leopold
Clinical Orthopaedics and Related Research,
University of Washington, Seattle, WA, USA

© Springer International Publishing AG 2018

19

C. Mauffrey, M.M. Scarlat (eds.), *Medical Writing and Research Methodology for the Orthopaedic Surgeon*, https://doi.org/10.1007/978-3-319-69350-7_4

find that successful research papers have several things in common. Papers that succeed in peer review:

- Ask focused, answerable research questions.
- Summarize their methods clearly.
- Present their results so the reader remembers them.
- Structure the introduction and discussion for maximum effect.
- Outline and justify the study's limitations.

4.3   Tips and Tricks for a Successful Submission

4.3.1   Ask Focused, Answerable Research Questions

Good research begins with good questions. To attract the attention of readers—a key mission of most journals—questions should be relevant to research or practice and should not have been answered definitively by earlier work. For the project to be practical, the questions must also be answerable within the means available: sufficient patient volume, financial and staff resources, equipment, and experience. Large studies, randomized or prospective studies, and blinded studies all increase the demands on the research team's experience and resources.

Clear questions focus on specific endpoints. Compare the following research questions:

"Is the risk of hip dislocation within 6 months of surgery greater in the direct anterior or the posterior approach to total hip arthroplasty?"

and

"What are the outcomes of direct anterior total hip arthroplasty?"

The former is an example of a clear question: In a single sentence, it describes the patient population, the intervention or exposure that will be studied, the comparator groups, and the outcome of greatest interest. A well-focused research question points to plausible methods that might be used to answer it (more on this just below) and gives the reader a clear expectation of what (s)he will gain by reading the study. The latter gives the reader no real inkling of what the study is about.

Vague terms like "outcomes" or "results" in general should be avoided in research questions, in favor of more specific, testable endpoints.

4.3.2   Summarize the Methods Clearly

Research questions that focus on specific questions help readers, but they also guide the research team to the right methods to answer them. Vague questions—like "what are the outcomes of direct anterior total hip arthroplasty?"—provide no such guidance. In this context, "outcomes" could refer to pain relief, return of function, the proportion of patients experiencing complications or undergoing reoperation, cost-effectiveness, or any of dozens of other more meaningful endpoints, each of which would call for entirely different study designs. Our better question—about early dislocations after surgery—can help the research team craft suitable methods to for arriving at the answers.

If the research design is particularly complicated, beginning a methods section with an overview paragraph that provides the "big picture" can be helpful. An experimental design figure can also sometimes help, if there are multiple experiments or modalities.

If the study asks several questions, as many do, there is nothing wrong—and a lot right—with topic sentences like "To test our first question [*restate question here*], we [*briefly summarize methods on how the first question was tested*]."

Good tools exist that can help the clinician-scientist present his or her methods clearly. The Centre for Evidence-Based Medicine has published multiple "Critical Appraisal Worksheets" for the common study designs: systematic review, diagnosis, prognosis, and therapy/RCT [1]. In these, an author can ensure that the methods presentation addresses the common sources of bias that readers care about in each of those study designs. They are briefly summarized below in Table 4.1.

In addition, three widely accepted and easy-to-use checklists walk authors through the most common types of clinical research studies. STROBE (Strengthening the Reporting of Observational Studies in Epidemiology) is handy for writing up retrospective clinical studies of many designs, including cohort, case control, and cross-sectional studies [2]. CONSORT (Consolidated Standards of Reporting

Table 4.1 Critically appraising clinical research methods

	Diagnostic study	Prognostic study	Therapy or RCT	Systematic review
Are the results valid?	Test evaluated in a representative spectrum of patients?	Patients assembled at a common (early) point in disease course?	Assignment of patients random?	What question did the systematic review address?
			Groups similar at start of trial?	
		Follow-up sufficiently long and complete?	Groups treated equally?	Unlikely that important, relevant studies were missed?
	Reference standard applied universally?	Outcome criteria objective or applied blindly?	All patients that entered the trial accounted for?	
		Adjustments made between subgroups?		Appropriate article inclusion criteria?
				Included studies valid for question?
	Independent, blind comparison between index and gold standard tests?		Measures objective or were patients and/or clinicians blinded?	Results similar from study to study?

(continued)

Table 4.1 (continued)

	Diagnostic study	Prognostic study	Therapy or RCT	Systematic review
What are the results?	Test characteristics presented? (sensitivity, specificity, positive predictive value, negative predictive value)	How likely are the events over time? [graph suggested]	How large was the treatment effect?	How were the results presented? [forest plot suggested]
		How precise are prognostic estimates?	What were the measures (RR, ARR, RRR, NNT)?	Heterogeneity explored?
			How precise was the estimate of treatment effect?	
Applicability of results?	Methods described in sufficient detail to permit replication?	Applicable to individual or group of patients?	Applicable to individual or group of patients?	Applicable to individual or group of patients?

Trials) walks the author through the key elements of randomized controlled trials [3]. Finally, PRISMA (Preferred Reporting Items for Systematic Reviews and Meta-analysis) covers what authors would want to know about the reporting of systematic reviews and meta-analysis [4]. Covering these in detail is beyond the scope of this chapter, but these tools are easy to use, comprehensive, and freely available on the Internet. In fact, their use is mandated by many better journals, including *The Journal of Bone and Joint Surgery* and *Clinical Orthopaedics and Related Research*.

4.3.3 Present the Results so the Reader Remembers Them

While every study design—indeed every study—will make different demands on its author in terms of how the results should be presented, the author should try not to make too many demands on the reader in the results section. After all, this is where the study's key messages get delivered, and the goal is to help the reader understand those messages. Several simple steps can help.

First, consider organizing the results section in parallel with the research questions. If there are three research questions or purposes, consider answering them with three results paragraphs, in the same order as those questions were posed. Remember, science is the process of answering questions. Presenting the questions and their answers in sequence makes it more likely the reader will retain those answers.

Next, rather than diving straight into complex analyses or statistics, begin each results paragraph with a plain language summary sentence that contains a minimum of jargon or names of statistical analyses. In fact, there is little reason to present the names of analyses at all in the results section, since they were already covered in methods. In this part of the paper, the reader wants the answers to the questions, not how those answers were derived.

Finally, focus on effect size and direction rather than "statistical significance." Again, the methods section should already have defined what the paper considers a statistical difference that was unlikely to have been a chance effect, and so the reader trusts that the author will not claim a "difference" that did not pass the relevant statistical test. In the results section, the reader simply wants know how large the difference was, and which treatment it favored.

For example, imagine a study that evaluated a new topical anticoagulant used during spine surgery by comparing it to placebo. Which topic sentence conveys more information?

When comparing Nobleedum spray to placebo, a significant difference was found on the t-test (p < 0.05).

or

Patients treated with Nobleedum spray experienced less blood loss during surgery than did patients treated with the placebo (850 ± 75 versus 400 ± 50 cm³, p = 0.02).

The second example is more effective because it identifies the endpoint being considered and gives the reader a sense both for the effect's size and its direction. It provides as much statistical information as the first example—in fact, more—but does so in a way that doesn't dwell on the unhelpful and often-confusing adjective "significant." Beginning each results paragraph with a clear topic sentence like that offered by the second example here makes it much more likely that the reader will understand and remember the study's main messages. In fact, the effective use of topic sentences allows the reader to discern a paper's main message quickly and easily, simply by reading the first sentence of each paragraph in the results section. Assume your readers are as busy as you are; make it easy on them.

4.3.4   Structure the Introduction and Discussion for Maximum Effect

We find that authors often are uncertain about what belongs in an introduction, what belongs in a discussion, and what doesn't belong in a paper at all. While every journal has its own house style—which includes not just formatting issues but also what kind of material goes in which section of the scientific papers it publishes—some general approaches serve well across the board. Here is one such approach:

Consider that the job of the introduction is to give the reader just enough information to allow him or her (1) to understand the importance of the topic, (2) to decide that reading on will be worth the time spent, and (3) to know precisely what questions the paper will answer. With that in mind, a short introduction— three paragraphs, one to meet each of those goals—usually does the trick in a straightforward clinical research paper. The first paragraph should convince the reader that the topic is important. While "important" will vary depending on who is reading (e.g., a great study on hallux valgus may not be important to a hand surgeon), in general an author can establish importance of a paper by convincing the reader that it addresses a problem that is common, morbid, expensive, or difficult to treat. The second paragraph should focus on the study's rationale: the gap in knowledge that the authors set out to fill when they decided to begin the project or a controversy that the study might help settle. A compelling rationale paragraph will convince the reader that staying with you is worth the time (s)he will need to invest, which is no small commitment. Simply saying that a topic has not been reported on before may not itself be a convincing rationale; sometimes, topics have not been explored because they are unimportant or uninteresting. This is why it is effective to begin with a paragraph of background (why the topic is important) before pointing to the study's rationale (the gaps in knowledge of that topic the study will help fill). Finally, end the introduction with a short paragraph consisting of the specific research questions or purposes. If the rationale paragraph is written clearly, the last paragraph on research questions indeed can consist only of "We therefore sought to study…" and provide the specific, testable research questions.

Short introductions do not mean bloated, discursive, or ill-focused discussions. An effective discussion will (1) hook the reader, (2) cover the study's limitations, (3) compare the findings to others, and (4) wrap it up. A discussion might open with a paragraph where the background and rationale are briefly restated, followed by a short summary of the paper's main findings (some journals prefer that the questions are restated instead of the main findings—check out the target journal for house style on this point). A discussion section must cover a study's limitations; whether this is done in the second paragraph of the discussion or toward the end of it is, once again, generally a matter of that journal's style. Next, consider organizing the discussion around the research questions. A paragraph of discussion per research question is a good place to start (if the question was important enough to ask, it's important enough to discuss)—and often a great place to stop, since more than this can result in a reader losing track of what is important. Each discussion paragraph should compare the findings on one research question to other studies on similar topics and speak to the generalizability of those findings; once again, it helps the reader if this is done in the order those questions were asked. If the study's results are different from others, the authors should suggest why this might be—different techniques? Different study populations? Different analytic methods? If the results are similar to those reported by others, the authors should explain how the new work extends what is known or why confirming it merits the reader's attention. Finally, a good discussion section should conclude by helping the reader know what might be done with the results, how (if at all) the findings should influence practice, what unanswered questions remain, and how future studies might go about answering them.

Anything more than that—exhaustive literature reviews, summaries of related laboratory research findings in clinical research papers, facts the team finds interesting and learned along the way—need not appear in a clinical research paper. Save those for the review article.

4.3.5 Outline and Justify the Study's Limitations

By the time a clinician-scientist is writing up a paper, (s)he has spent months or years living with the project. Emotional bonds form. But like our friends and relatives—and like us—our papers have limitations. Good papers discuss these candidly. Simply listing a study's limitations, though, is not helpful; the goal of this section of the discussion is to justify those limitations, that is, to help the reader understand how each specific limitation influences the effect size, generalizability, or robustness of the main findings. A good way to do this is to focus on the main kinds of bias that commonly influence the research design that was used; the Centre for Evidence-Based Medicine offers some useful outlines of these topics [1]. Here, we will focus on three of the most common kinds of bias that influence the conclusion in the most common research design in orthopedic journals: the retrospective study on therapy [5]. Three kinds of bias beset papers of this design in almost all instances: selection bias, transfer bias, and assessment bias [6]. In retrospective observational studies, readers are concerned about these kinds of bias, and authors should help them understand to what degree the conclusions are compromised by them.

Selection Bias: Do the study's patients truly represent the patient population of interest, or were only the "easy ones" studied? In general, the effect of this kind of bias is to inflate the apparent benefits of newer treatments being studied.

Transfer Bias: Was the follow-up sufficiently long and complete to identify the outcomes (and complications or failures) of interest? As patients who are missing are more likely to have had an adverse event—failure, complication, or reoperation—the higher the proportion of patients lost to follow-up, the better the treatment being studied will look [7, 8]. A study reporting good results in 95% of patients but accounting for only 60% of the patients treated may indeed be misleading. This is especially important if the treatment groups suffered from differential loss to follow-up; if the treatment group has lost more patients to follow-up than the control group, the treatment will look better than it probably is.

Assessment Bias: Who assessed the outcomes, and how were they assessed? The answer to a well-constructed research question can be undermined or invalidated by improperly assessing the answers to that question. Assessment bias can occur when an interested party (e.g., the operating surgeon) performs the outcome measure assessments or if non-validated tools are used. Be especially mindful of studies that purport to assess "satisfaction"; this is notoriously difficult to evaluate [9].

4.4 Common Mistakes and How to Prevent Them

- *Don't ask vague research questions.* Avoid terms like "outcomes," "results," and "our experiences with," in favor of more specific study endpoints. Using the Centre for Evidence-Based Medicine's "PICO" tool (Patient, Intervention, Comparison, Outcome) can help, as well [10].

- *Don't confuse statistical significance and clinical importance.* There is little benefit—and much potential harm [11] to using the terms "significant" or "statistically significant" anyplace other than the statistical methods section of a paper. Readers who are not statistically savvy risk confusing the passing of a statistical test with the clinical importance of a finding. Some results are "statistically significant" because the study group is very large—indeed this is common with large randomized trials and national databases or registries—even though the effect sizes are small. Make no claims of difference unless those differences indeed have cleared the statistical hurdles set in the method's section, but once a difference has cleared that hurdle, focus on whether the observed difference is clinically meaningful. In the results section, concentrate instead on effect size, odds or hazard ratios, numbers needed to treat or harm, and other measures that allow the reader an intuitive sense for whether the observed differences were large or small. Consider framing the results in terms of the minimum clinically important difference (MCID), if it is known for the outcomes tool being used [12] and explain what it means if the observed "differences" indeed are smaller than the MCID, as this can completely change a study's conclusion. In the discussion section, indicate whether those observed differences are worth the inevitable trade-offs that arise in clinical medicine, like cost, risk, and uncertainty.
- *Don't waste your time—read the author instructions.* Read a journal's author instructions before submitting (or even writing up) your work for that journal. Make sure your work is within that journal's remit and that you've adhered to that journal's house style. Many journals offer templates that make writing to their style easier. Since their reviewers have grown accustomed to seeing manuscripts in that style, not adhering to it places your work at a severe competitive disadvantage in the review process.
- *Don't violate normative or ethical standards of scientific publishing.* Each journal has its own standards for such things as authorship, conflicts of interest, and redundancy; many better journals employ available and well-considered international standards, such as those articulated by the International Committee of Medical Journal Editors [13] and the Committee on Publication Ethics [14]. Be familiar with the journal's policies on these matters before submitting, familiarize yourself with the available guidelines and tools at www.icmje.org and www. publicationethics.org, and adhere to them. If in doubt, email your query to the journal's editor. Ghost or guest authorship, undisclosed or incorrectly disclosed conflicts of interest, and redundant publication ("salami slicing") will commonly result in a manuscript's rejection or worse. Errors in these areas can taint or ruin careers.
- *Don't overreach—present your conclusions modestly.* Few things turn a reader (or reviewer or editor) off more than an immodest or overstated conclusion. If you are uncertain about whether your study's conclusion paints within the lines, consider reading your paper to someone whom you know disagrees with your study's point of view, and be open to modifying things accordingly, since there is a good chance that one or more reviewers may not see things exactly as you do.

4.5   Take-Home Messages

- *Good science is about questions and their answers.* Ask clear, focused questions around specific, testable endpoints. Organize every section of the paper—methods, results, and discussion—around those questions.
- *Make sure your reader knows how the questions were tested.* Use STROBE, CONSORT, or PRISMA (whichever applies) to structure a methods section that is robust and easy to follow. Reassure the reader that the common kinds of bias identified in the Centre for Evidence-Based Medicine's "Critical Appraisal" tools [1] are not disqualifying flaws.
- *Present the results so simply that no one can misunderstand them.* Begin each results paragraph with a plain language summary sentence that a nonscientist would understand. Focus on the endpoint tested, the effect's size, and its direction, not "statistical significance."
- *Hook the reader with a background that demonstrates the study's importance and a rationale that convinces him/her that (s)he cannot afford to skip over the paper.* These elements are the "meat" of the introduction section and should appear again in the first paragraph of the discussion.
- *Be modest.* Present the study's limitations explicitly, and you make it clear how those limitations should influence the reader's understanding of the study's main findings. Indicate to the reader to what degree the work might—or might not—generalize to other patient groups or practice setting. Focus the conclusions on what was actually tested.

Acknowledgment The authors gratefully acknowledge Richard A. Brand, MD, whose efforts to refine and disseminate a question-driven approach to scientific reporting deeply influenced our own approaches and whose paper "Writing for *Clinical Orthopaedics and Related Research*" [15] is a must read, regardless of what journal one is writing for.

References

1. Oxford Centre for Evidence- Based Medicine. Critical appraisal tools. http://www.cebm.net/critical-appraisal/. Accessed 22 June 2015.
2. von Elm E, Altman DG, Egger M, Pocock SJ, Gøtzsche PC, Vandenbroucke JP, STROBE Initiative. The Strengthening the Reporting of Observational Studies in Epidemiology (STROBE) statement: guidelines for reporting observational studies. J Clin Epidemiol. 2008;61(4):344–9.
3. Schulz KF, Altman DG, Moher D, CONSORT Group. CONSORT 2010 statement: updated guidelines for reporting parallel group randomised trials. Ann Intern Med. 2010;152:726.
4. Moher D, Liberati A, Tetzlaff J, Altman DG, The PRISMA Group. Preferred reporting items for systematic reviews and meta-analyses: the PRISMA statement. Ann Intern Med. 2009;151(4):264.
5. Wupperman R, Davis R, Obremskey WT. Level of evidence in Spine compared to other orthopedic journals. Spine. 2007;32(3):388–93.
6. Leopold SS. Editorial: let's talk about level IV: the bones of a good restrospective case series. Clin Orthop Relat Res. 2013;471(2):353–4.

7. Paradis C. Bias in surgical research. Ann Surg. 2008;248(2):180–8.
8. Pannucci C, Wilkins E. Identifying and avoiding bias in research. Plast Reconstr Surg. 2010;126(2):619–25.
9. Ring D, Leopold SS. Editorial: measuring satisfaction: can it be done? Clin Orthop Relat Res. 2015;473(10):3071–3.
10. Oxford Centre for Evidence- Based Medicine. Asking focused questions. http://www.cebm.net/asking-focused-questions/. Accessed 22 June 2015.
11. Leopold SS. Editorial: words and meaning in scientific reporting: consecutive, prospective, and significant. Clin Orthop Relat Res. 2013;471(9):2731–2.
12. Schiffer G. CORR insights: the minimum clinically important difference of patient-rated wrist evaluation score for patients with distal radius fractures. Clin Orthop Relat Res. 2015;473(10):3242–4.
13. International Committee of Medical Journal Editors. Defining the role of authors and contributors. 2014. http://www.icmje.org/recommendations/browse/roles-and-responsibilities/defining-the-role-of-authors-and-contributors.html. Accessed 21 June 2015.
14. Committee on Publication Ethics. Guidelines. http://publicationethics.org/resources/guidelines. Accessed 29 Sept 2015.
15. Brand RA. Editorial: writing for clinical orthopaedics and related research. Clin Orthop Relat Res. 2008;466:239–47.

Medical Writing: Systematic Reviews and Meta-analyses

5

Simon Tiziani and Hans-Christoph Pape

5.1 Introduction

5.1.1 Historical Aspects

Until three decades ago, access to medical knowledge represented a major limiting factor, on one hand. Medical books were priced highly, so that they were limited to larger libraries, or wealthy individuals. On the other hand, these textbooks tended to be out of date rather quickly, and there were difficulties in keeping up with the rapidly growing body of knowledge in due time.

In contrast, we nowadays tend to struggle with the sheer amount of publications being released daily, rather than issues in accessibility. This applies for global knowledge and information relevant for medical subspecialties. Specifically, the growing body of open-access publishing has led to a rapid turnover and quick accessibility in that regard [1].

5.1.2 Issues in Obtaining Medical Information Today

It has long been recognized that even particular clinical research questions are difficult to answer sufficiently through a single study. As of today, randomized controlled trials are considered the gold standard for study designs aimed at answering questions about the efficacy of a new medical treatment. However, even those randomized controlled trials that are supposed to have been conducted under high-quality circumstances are known to have limitations. Some authors suggested that sample sizes are too small; others discussed the presence of a persisting bias innate to the respective study designs. Furthermore, the applicability of the obtained results

S. Tiziani (✉) • H.-C. Pape
Department of Trauma, University of Zurich, Zurich, Switzerland
e-mail: simon.tiziani@usz.ch

© Springer International Publishing AG 2018
C. Mauffrey, M.M. Scarlat (eds.), *Medical Writing and Research Methodology for the Orthopaedic Surgeon*, https://doi.org/10.1007/978-3-319-69350-7_5

to the general population has been questioned. Nonetheless, physicians, politicians, and the media frequently emphasize the results obtained by one particular study—despite the fact that its relevance may be limited.

Moreover, the number of manuscripts published in medicine and biomedical research continues to increase. Thereby, it becomes progressively difficult even for a specialist in his respective field to stay up-to-date with his/her current particular research area. This applies even more for general practitioners that are bound to cover multiple medical fields. For these, it has become impossible to stay up-to-date with the literature.

The aim of this chapter is to give the reader an overview on how to critically read, plan, and report about the current literature. Specifically, it deals with the information gathered in systematic reviews and/or meta-analyses. Furthermore, we try to equip the reader with the crucial references to guidelines on the conduction and reporting of such projects.

5.1.3 The Development of Systematic Reviews and Meta-Analyses

Systematic reviews and meta-analyses became available in the 1970s. They were closely related with the ability to use digital data and compare large trials and sets of data. These reviews tried to summarize those that appeared to gather too much information to be overseen by individuals or groups of researchers. Therefore, the idea of a systematic review became to provide a systematic collection of all research conducted and published regarding a specific research question.

The strategy of summarizing existing studies was fostered by Dr. A. Cochrane, who recognized that bigger data analyses are central to new developments in medical research. His monograph *Effectiveness and Efficiency* was published in 1971 and delivered a scathing criticism of medical research and of solely looking at randomized controlled trials for answers. He called for systematic reviews in order to provide evidence-based knowledge. Eventually, this led to the foundation of the "The Cochrane Collaboration" in 1993 with the goal to "prepare, maintain, and disseminate systematic reviews of the effects of health care interventions" [2]. The *Cochrane Library* contains the *Cochrane Database on Systematic Reviews and provided a major advancement of evidence by gathering* of systematic reviews and meta-analysis in a major way [3].

Following the development of systematic reviews, meta-analyses were designed to synthesize results from different studies that looked at the same question in the same manner. The goal was to provide a quantitative pooled estimate and thus support or deny current evidence. In this line, meta-analyses can be but do not always have to represent part of a systematic review [4].

It is understood that any systemic review and meta-analysis can be vulnerable to bias, as it has to rely on the input of the data summarized in a given study. Therefore, a key task for researchers that deal with these studies is to test whether data are reported incorrectly and whether key information regarding the included studies is missing [5].

5.1.4   Reading and Reviewing a Systematic Review and Meta-Analysis

It is vital to assess the information that lead to a systematic review. Moreover, systematic reviews should also be critically read an evaluated for their clinical applicability. Guidelines have been described to improve the quality for reading a systematic review and meta-analysis published in 2014 [6]. In these guidelines, the authors state that ideally, *two judgments* should be made before applying the results to patient care. Every judgment includes different questions the reader should know that are listed in their original form below.

The *first judgment* regards credibility of the methods of the systematic review. Among the questions to be answered are the following ones:

- Did the review address sensible clinical question?
- Was the research for relevant studies exhaustive?
- Were selection and assessment of studies reproducible?
- Did the review present results that are ready for clinical application?
- Did the review address confidence in estimates of effects?

The last point is crucial because subsequent criteria used for the second judgment can't be evaluated without knowing whether the authors reported on the different bias found in the included studies. Also, heterogeneity of the body of evidence is an issue. The *second judgment* includes six relevant points and is designed to test the confidence in the effect estimates. This reflects whether the reported effects correspond to the true effects and whether they are expected to be toppled by future studies:

- How serious is the risk of bias in the body of evidence?
- Are the results consistent across studies?
- How precise are the results?
- Do the results directly apply to my patient?
- Is there concern about reporting bias?
- Are there reasons to increase confidence rating?

5.2   Planning a Systematic Review and Meta-Analysis

As with every research project, systematic reviews and meta-analysis have to be planned carefully and then be conducted diligently. There are numerous articles and books that deal with the planning and execution of systematic results. It is our goal to give a short summary of the most important points one should adhere to when planning a systematic review. The process of a systematic review should follow the basic steps listed below [4, 6]:

1. Formulate the question to be investigated and define eligibility criteria.
2. Search for trials.
3. Screen titles and abstracts for eligibility

Fig. 5.1 Hierarchy of evidence

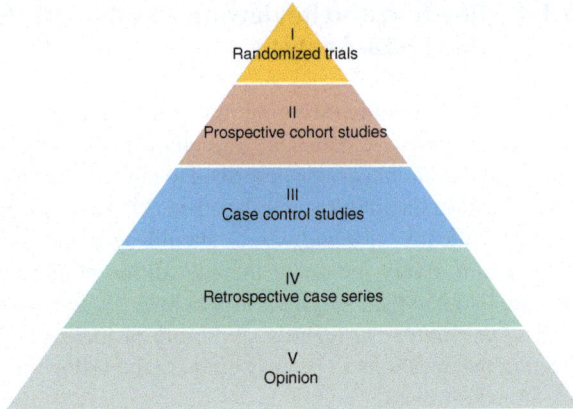

4. Read full texts of possibly eligible trials to determine their methodological quality, and justify exclusions.
5. Assess the risk of bias.
6. Compile data from trials included.
7. Analyze the obtained trials, and apply statistical synthesis by conducting a meta-analysis if possible.
8. Critically report your findings.

It appears that two major pitfalls should be considered when conducting a systematic review: (1) incomplete search for trials only via one search portal and (2) inclusion of trials in the systematic review only reading the abstract.

Thus, the goal of a systematic review is to adequately display and interpret the currently available body of evidence regarding a medical question. This however is contingent on the fact that all available literature is assessed for eligibility. An exclusive search on PubMed does not match the current needs of evidence (Fig. 5.1). In addition to the routine searches of Medline and Embase, investigators should also consider clinical trial registries, foreign language publications, non-peer-reviewed journals, and unpublished information known to physicians in the respective fields.

5.3 Reporting Systematic Reviews and Meta-Analysis

As important as carefully conducting the systematic review is the correct reporting of obtained results. A review of conducted systematic reviews shows that quality of reporting is still subject to vast variability with investigator not reporting key information (e.g., whether there was an assessment of bias in the body of evidence). It is also interesting to see that quality varies between Cochrane and non-Cochrane reviews, with Cochrane reviews showing significantly better reporting [7].

Parallel to the CONSORT guidelines for reporting randomized controlled trials, an effort was made to define guidelines for reporting systematic reviews which led to the publication of the QUORUM guideline (quality of reporting of meta-analysis) in 1999 [8]. The guidelines later were revised and published as the PRISMA criteria (Preferred Reporting Items for Systematic reviews and Meta-analysis) in 2009 [5]. PRISMA allows investigator to follow a step-by-step checklist when reporting their results in the form of a systematic review. The checklist includes 27 items to guide the author through manuscript compilation. An explanation of each recommendation is provided including an example.

One of the frequent flaws when trying to publish a systematic review is the failure of adhering to reporting standards. Incomplete reporting impairs the inability to assess the review according the selected criteria. It is of no use if possible bias of the body of evidence was investigated and taken under consideration when reporting about it is lacking.

Another pitfall is over-interpretation and hyping. Conclusions should be limited to the scope of the results yielded by the review and considering the limitations of the review itself. As often a systematic review is seen as the tool to correct for such bias in randomized controlled trials, one has to be extra careful with making definite statements and recommendations and be sure of the evidence supporting them [9].

Currently, different systems for confidence ratings have been described. According to the GRADE (Grading of Recommendations Assessment, Development and Evaluation) criteria, the clinical evidence levels can be categorized into high, moderate, low, and very low [10].

5.4 Big Data

Another approach to overcome bias and to try to get as close to the real truth is connected with the term "big data" which has seen a rise in popularity lately. Clinical research often presents with the problem of being underpowered. Either a sample size calculation was omitted while planning the study or the calculated sample size is so big that a study would not be feasible. This especially applies to studies trying to investigate an event of which the prevalence already is low and supposed relative changes due to an intervention are low as well. It is not uncommon for a sample size calculation to kill a project.

Studies about postoperative infection rates after spinal surgery may be a good example. With the infection rates, depending on the procedure and the reason for operation, being in the single digits, studies assessing a change in postoperative infection rates would have to include patients in the thousands. For most ideas or interventions, this is simply not warranted.

The abovementioned facts often lead to researchers ignoring sample size calculations or even choosing not to conduct one to begin with. An underpowered study can be tainted by unknown bias, and usually significance cannot be detected, or obtained results cannot be generalized to the general population.

Thus, big data can be seen as an effort to deal with the abovementioned problems. It can take different forms. On the one hand, the most commonly associated with big data may be nationwide registries (TARN, DGU, Japanese registry, NTDB). Big data is not limited to registry and encompasses large cohort studies or randomized controlled trials with big patient collectives. Large data sets require specific handling. The vast amount of data especially in registries is prone to selection bias, and if a database reaches a certain size, every analysis with standard day-to-day statistical tools produces significant differences. This is why the maintenance and interpretation of big registry requires a professional team including biostaticians [11].

References

1. Bastian H, Glasziou P, Chalmers I. Seventy-five trials and eleven systematic reviews a day: how will we ever keep up? PLoS Med. 2010;7(9):e1000326.
2. Levin A. The Cochrane Collaboration. Ann Intern Med. 2001;135(4):309–12.
3. Shah HM, Chung KC. Archie Cochrane and his vision for evidence-based medicine. Plast Reconstr Surg. 2009;124(3):982–8.
4. Greenhalgh T. Papers that summarise other papers (systematic reviews and meta-analyses). BMJ. 1997;315(7109):672–5.
5. Liberati A, Altman DG, Tetzlaff J, Mulrow C, Gotzsche PC, Ioannidis JP, Clarke M, Devereaux PJ, Kleijnen J, Moher D. The PRISMA statement for reporting systematic reviews and meta-analyses of studies that evaluate healthcare interventions: explanation and elaboration. BMJ. 2009;339:b2700.
6. Murad MH, Montori VM, Ioannidis JP, Jaeschke R, Devereaux PJ, Prasad K, Neumann I, Carrasco-Labra A, Agoritsas T, Hatala R, et al. How to read a systematic review and meta-analysis and apply the results to patient care: users' guides to the medical literature. JAMA. 2014;312(2):171–9.
7. Moher D, Tetzlaff J, Tricco AC, Sampson M, Altman DG. Epidemiology and reporting characteristics of systematic reviews. PLoS Med. 2007;4(3):e78.
8. Moher D, Cook DJ, Eastwood S, Olkin I, Rennie D, Stroup DF. Improving the quality of reports of meta-analyses of randomised controlled trials: the QUOROM statement. Quality of reporting of meta-analyses. Lancet. 1999;354(9193):1896–900.
9. McInnes MD, Bossuyt PM. Pitfalls of systematic reviews and meta-analyses in imaging research. Radiology. 2015;277(1):13–21.
10. Guyatt GH, Oxman AD, Vist GE, Kunz R, Falck-Ytter Y, Alonso-Coello P, Schunemann HJ. GRADE: an emerging consensus on rating quality of evidence and strength of recommendations. BMJ. 2008;336(7650):924–6.
11. Slobogean GP, Giannoudis PV, Frihagen F, Forte ML, Morshed S, Bhandari M. Bigger data, bigger problems. J Orthop Trauma. 2015;29(Suppl 12):S43–6.

Epidemiological Studies

Charles M. Court-Brown and Stuart A. Aitken

Epidemiology has been defined as the 'study of the distribution and determinants of disease frequency' in human populations. In their excellent book on *Epidemiology in Medicine*, Hennekens et al. [1] state that epidemiology may be viewed as based on two fundamental assumptions. Firstly, that human disease does not occur at random and secondly that human disease has causal and preventative measures that can be identified through systematic investigation of different populations or subgroups of individuals within a population in different places or at different times. Major areas of epidemiological study include the aetiology, transmission and screening of disease and investigations of the effects of treatment, these often being undertaken in prospective randomised studies.

We have attempted to define the role of epidemiological investigations in orthopaedic surgery. We will present the types of epidemiological studies that can be undertaken and a basic analysis of how the results of these studies can be assessed. This chapter is aimed at clinicians, and therefore we will not cover the whole of epidemiology. If further information is required, a specialist medical epidemiology [1] text should be consulted. As both authors have a major interest in orthopaedic trauma, most of the examples of the use of epidemiological studies and calculations will be related to fractures. However, the principles outlined in this chapter can be used for many diseases and medical conditions. An outline of the aims of an epidemiological study is shown in Table 6.1.

C.M. Court-Brown (✉)
Department of Orthopaedic Trauma, University of Edinburgh, Edinburgh, UK
e-mail: ccb@courtbrown.com

S.A. Aitken
Department of Orthopaedic Trauma, MaineGeneral Medical Center, Augusta, ME, US

© Springer International Publishing AG 2018
C. Mauffrey, M.M. Scarlat (eds.), *Medical Writing and Research Methodology for the Orthopaedic Surgeon*, https://doi.org/10.1007/978-3-319-69350-7_6

Table 6.1 The basic principles of conducting an epidemiological study

1. Establish that a problem exists that needs investigation
2. Collect as much information as possible about the disease or medical condition that you wish to investigate. Look for factors that predispose patients to the condition and factors that increase or decrease the likelihood of getting the condition
3. Look for patterns and trends that may identify risk factors for getting the condition
4. Formulate a hypothesis and test it
5. Publish the results

6.1 History

It has been stated that Hippocrates theorised in the fifth century BC that the development of human disease might be related to the external environment as well as to the individual environment of a patient [1]. He suggested that the seasons, weather, local environment and the patient's occupation and exercise regime might affect their tendency to develop different diseases. He believed that sickness of the human body was caused by an imbalance of the four humours: black bile, yellow bile, phlegm and blood. When these humours were in balance, the patient was healthy, but when they were out of balance, disease occurred. This belief led to the use of bloodletting and dieting in medicine. He devised the terms endemic, for diseases confined to one location, and epidemic, for diseases seen at a particular time.

There was no apparent attempt made to measure the impact of external stimuli on disease or mortality until 1662 when John Graunt published *The Nature and Political Observations Made Upon the Bills of Mortality*. He analysed the weekly reports of births and deaths in London and, for the first time, quantified patterns of disease in a population. He recorded a higher birth rate and mortality in males than females, a high infant mortality and a seasonal variation in mortality.

Hennekens et al. [1] documented that little further progress was made until William Farr was given responsibility for medical statistics in the Office of the Registrar General for England and Wales in 1839. He set up a system for recording the numbers and causes of death, and he also analysed mortality in different occupations. However, it would seem that his major contribution was to facilitate the work of John Snow, the physician who postulated that cholera was transmitted by contaminated water. Snow's work revolutionised epidemiological analysis of disease. As the treatment of infectious diseases improved, epidemiological analysis was used more in chronic diseases.

Semmelweiss was also an important pioneer in medical epidemiology. In 1847 he studied and reduced infant mortality in a hospital in Vienna by instituting a disinfection procedure. As is often the case in medicine, his colleagues did not appreciate the progress that he had made, and disinfection was not widely practiced until the work of Joseph Lister was accepted. In more recent times, the work of Doll and Hill [2] drew attention to the association of smoking and lung cancer.

The assumption is often made that epidemiological analysis of fractures is a recent phenomenon. However, surgeons in the nineteenth century undertook epidemiological analysis of the fractures that they saw. Malgaigne [3] undertook two analyses of fracture epidemiology between 1806–1808 and 1830–1839. He examined 2377 fractures and analysed the age and gender of the patients, as well as the seasonality and location of the fractures. He stated that fractures were commonly seen in patients between 25 and 60 years of age, but that there were very few patients older than 60 years. He thought that fractures were more commonly seen in spring and that diaphyseal fractures were seen in adulthood, but intraarticular fractures were seen in the elderly. He also recognised that fractures of the 'cervix femoris' and 'cervix humeri' occurred in old age and that fractures of the 'carpal extremity of the radius' occurred in women.

Gurtl [3] analysed 1383 fractures in 1862 and drew attention to the fact that the highest incidence of fractures occurred in patients aged ≥60 years but that only 8.5% of his patients were in this age group. Stimson [3] defined the distribution of fractures in New York between 1894 and 1903 and showed that the prevalence of the fractures was largely determined by the season.

In more recent years, there has been an increased interest in the epidemiology of fractures, particularly in fractures of the elderly as they are becoming very common and are expensive to treat. A number of techniques have been used to study the epidemiology of fractures, and these highlight the different techniques that can be used and some of their drawbacks.

6.2   Types of Study

The types of study that are often used in epidemiological analysis are listed in Table 6.2. There are two basic types, these being descriptive and analytical studies. Descriptive epidemiological studies assess the distribution of diseases or conditions such as fractures. They assess which populations develop the condition and how the frequency of the condition varies with time and other parameters. Analytic epidemiological studies test the conclusions of descriptive investigations as to whether a particular factor causes or prevents the condition being studied. An example of these study types is the initial descriptive report of the epidemiology of all non-spinal fractures in a defined population in Scotland in 2010/2011 [4] with reference to gender and age (Fig. 6.1a) and a later analytical study of whether social deprivation increased or decreased the incidence of fractures encountered [5] (Fig. 6.1b). The secondary analysis of the original descriptive study showed that social deprivation was associated with an increased incidence of fractures in the most deprived 10% of the population.

Table 6.2 Types of epidemiological studies

Descriptive studies	Analytical studies
Correlational studies	Observational studies
Case reports	Case-control studies
Case series	Cohort studies
Cross-sectional surveys	Interventional studies

Fig. 6.1 (**a**) Descriptive study of the age and gender of patients with a fracture in a defined population over a 1-year period [4]. (**b**) Analysis of the effect of the social decile of the patients on the incidence of fractures [5]. Decile 1 is most affluent and Decile 10 is least affluent

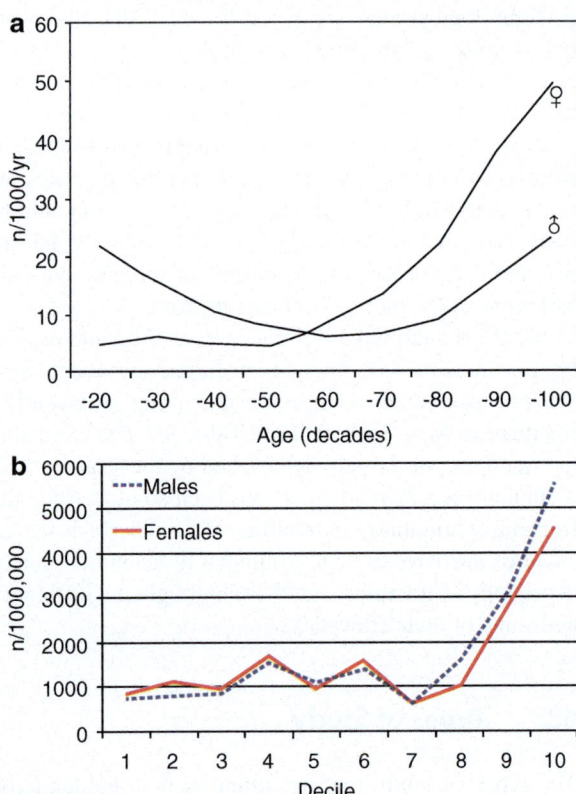

6.3   Descriptive Studies

Descriptive epidemiology is mainly concerned with the general characteristics of a disease or condition. Usually fairly basic descriptions are analysed. In fracture epidemiology these would usually include demographical patient data (e.g. age, gender, marital status, occupation) and information regarding the type of fracture. The particular value of descriptive studies is that they often provide the first evidence of the cause of a disease or medical condition. In orthopaedic research analysis of the distribution of osseous tumours, inflammatory joint disease or other bone diseases may well help determine the cause of these various conditions.

There are three types of descriptive studies (Table 6.2). These are correlational studies, case reports or case series and cross-sectional surveys.

6.4   Correlational Studies

In correlational studies data on large, hopefully entire, populations are used to describe the condition in relation to factors of particular interest. Two recent examples of orthopaedic correlational studies are *An Analysis of the use of Anti-Rheumatic*

Drugs in Rheumatoid Surgery [6] and *An Analysis of the role of Physical Activity in Preventing Falls and Subsequent Injury in Middle Aged Adults* [7]. In the first study 11,333 patients from Quebec's physician billing and hospitalisation database between 2002 and 2011 were analysed. The conclusion of the study was that longer exposure to antirheumatic drugs within the first year after diagnosis of rheumatoid arthritis was associated with a longer time to joint replacement surgery [6].

In the second study a much larger population was used. The US Behavioural Risk Factor Surveillance System in 2010 was analysed. The authors examined the number of adults aged ≥45 years who reported falls in the previous 3 months, and they questioned the participants about the injuries that the falls had caused. They found that of the 340,680 participants, 70.7% reported engaging in leisure time physical activity. These active participants experienced fewer falls and fewer fall-related injuries, the inference being that falls prevention interventions could be developed [7].

An advantage of correlational studies is that they are relatively easy to undertake provided the database exists. Governments and private health agencies routinely collect information, and, provided one can be sure that their information is representative of the whole population, good results can be obtained. However, surgeons should be aware that private health insurance company databases do not contain information about the whole population, and analysis of the results is likely to highlight socioeconomic differences in the population, as insured people tend to be more affluent.

A disadvantage of correlational studies is that one is often not able to identify whether the disease or condition being studied is associated with a particular subsection of the population. In addition, it is difficult to control for confounding factors. Hypothetically, one might demonstrate that dietary inadequacy is associated with a bone condition, but this, in fact, may simply represent socioeconomic deprivation or some other factor that is responsible for the condition being studied. A correlational study can raise a hypothesis, which can then be investigated with an analytical study. An example is shown in Fig. 6.1 where the possibility of an association between fractures and deprivation was raised after the results of the initial correlational study were available. In addition, correlational data provide average population results rather than highlighting which subsection of the population is at risk. If the relationship between a condition and a possible cause is not linear, it is unlikely to be shown by a correlational study.

6.5   Case Reports and Case Series

It is often stated that case reports and case series represent an important interface between clinical medicine and epidemiology. They describe a single patient or a group of patients with a similar condition. Their main use is to help identify new conditions or complications so that the physician or surgeon can be educated and take appropriate action.

Case reports are relatively common, and, while interesting, they do not often alter medical practice. Within the last 10 years or so, many case reports have simply been a reason to carry out a systematic review of the literature associated with the particular condition being presented. Analysis of the recent literature shows that case reports remain popular. It is impossible to know how useful modern case reports will be in the future, but two recently published case reports that might prove useful to surgeons are *Subtrochanteric Femoral Fracture in a Child after Removal of Femoral Neck Screws* [8] and *Atraumatic Bilateral Femoral Neck Fracture in a Premenopausal Female with Hypovitaminosis D* [9].

In contrast, case series can be useful in providing surgeons with information about a relatively rare condition. The presentation of more than one case may allow a hypothesis to be made rather than merely studying a single case of interest. A good example of this is the association with AIDS and homosexuality. Five cases of unusual pneumonia were reported in 1981 [10], and this paper helped to define a new problem and to initiate wider study. As with case reports, it is impossible to know which recently published case series may change medical practice, but two recent reports are of interest. One documents three insufficiency fractures following radiation of soft tissue tumours [11], and the other describes five cases of vertebral compression fracture as the initial presentation of amyloidosis [12]. The authors point out that there seems to be an association of vertebral compression fractures with liver involvement in amyloidosis. Case reports and case series are interesting and may well be influential, but they cannot be used to test a statistical association.

6.6   Cross-Sectional Surveys

The last type of descriptive study is a cross-sectional survey, also known as a prevalence survey. In this type of study, a disease or medical condition is assessed in a well-defined population and is usually carried out for a defined time period, often 1 year. These surveys provide an assessment of the frequency of a disease or condition in a population at a specific time. This type of study can be used to produce information about the causality of a condition, such as fractures. Cross-sectional surveys are very useful in defining the fractures that occur following motor vehicle accidents, sports injuries and standing falls.

An example of information gained from a cross-sectional study is shown in Table 6.3. This shows the epidemiology of different modes of injury that resulted in non-spinal fractures, in a 1-year study of a defined population in Edinburgh, Scotland [4]. It immediately allows one to know that 62.5% of fractures occurred as a result of a fall from a standing height and that 70% occurred in females. Only 5.2% of fractures occurred as a result of motor vehicle accidents, but the prevalence of multiple fractures and open fractures as a result of motor vehicle accidents was relatively high. This type of study facilitates planning of medical resources and allows surgeons to anticipate the spectrum of injuries they are likely to encounter, locally and elsewhere in regions with similar population demographics.

When undertaking this type of cross-sectional study, one should be careful to undertake it over an appropriate time period. Hypothetically, if the results shown in Table 6.3 had been undertaken over a 3-month period in winter, one might have had

Table 6.3 The results of a cross-sectional study [4] investigating how different fractures are caused

	Prevalence (%)	Incidence (n/10⁵/year)	Average age (years)			Older patients		Fracture types		M/F
			All	Male	Female	≥65 years	≥80 years	Multiple	Open	
Standing fall	62.5	836.4	62.3	54.3	65.7	38.9	20.6	1.5	0.5	30/70
Low fall	4.2	57.9	51.7	48.2	55.2	27.1	10.8	6.8	3.1	51/49
Fall (height)	2.3	31.6	36.0	37.5	30.0	8.1	2.5	33.0	10.6	88/12
Blow/assault	13.6	182.6	33.3	31.1	40.1	3.6	1.0	5.7	5.8	75/25
Sport	11.1	149.2	31.3	30.4	35.5	3.0	0.3	2.1	0.6	82/18
MVA	5.2	69.6	42.6	41.7	45.8	10.2	3.0	17.4	6.4	78/22
Pathological	0.4	4.8	67.3	63.5	70.3	60.0	24.0	0	0	44/56
Spontaneous	0.3	2.7	49.9	44.5	54.0	21.4	21.4	0	0	43/57

This type of study facilitates planning and allocation of resources as well as informing surgeons about their patients a different prevalence of sports injuries and possibly a higher prevalence of falls in the elderly. Thus one should take care to use an appropriate time period. The other problem that relates to cross-sectional studies is the difficulty of standardising the population used in the study. The patients in the study shown in Table 6.3 were from a defined area where only one hospital treats fractures [4]. This, however, is rare, and, especially in large towns, it is difficult to accurately assess the incidence and prevalence of fractures if patients can go to two or three different hospitals. These difficulties will be discussed later in this chapter.

6.7   Analytical Studies

In analytical studies a group of individuals is examined to see if the likelihood of disease or of having a particular medical condition is determined by being exposed to a particular factor or stimulus. Thus in orthopaedic trauma, one might analyse a group of middle-aged and elderly females to see if the incidence of femoral diaphyseal fractures was affected by the administration of bisphosphonates. There are two types of analytical studies, these being observational and interventional studies. The difference is in the role of the investigator. In observational studies the investigator observes the course of events and merely records who has been exposed to the potentially causative stimulus or variable that is being studied and who has developed the disease or condition of interest. In interventional studies the investigator introduces a potentially influential variable and then observes the patients to determine whether the occurrence or course of the disease or condition is affected.

6.8   Observational Studies

There are two types of observational studies, the case-control study and cohort study. In a case-control study, a series of patients who have the disease or condition under investigation (cases) are compared with an equivalent group of people who do not (controls), on the assumption that prior exposure to some identifiable attribute or event has led to the development of the disease in the former. The proportion of patients exposed to the causative factor or event in the cases and control groups is then analysed. A recent example of this type of study is that of Bishop et al. [13], who retrospectively analysed risk factors contributing to knee stiffness after periarticular fracture. The authors compared a series of fracture patients with knee stiffness that required treatment with a similarly injured group of patients without knee stiffness. They found that exposure to certain injury factors (extensor mechanism disruption, requirement for fasciotomies and wounds requiring flap coverage) contributed to the development of knee stiffness after a periarticular knee fracture.

In cohort studies the subjects being analysed are divided into two groups depending on whether they have been exposed to a particular factor or stimulus. They are then followed for a specific time period to define whether they develop the condition under investigation. These are usually protracted investigations that last many years, depending on the natural history and progression of the disease of interest. It is also important to realise that the term 'cohort study' is widely misused in orthopaedic surgery. It has come to mean a large cohort of subjects, whereas many cohort studies are actually correlational studies or cross-sectional studies. A recent orthopaedic example of a cohort study was published by Teng et al. [14]. This was in fact a meta-analysis of six cohort studies looking at the effect of smoking on prostheses-related complications after total hip arthroplasty. They showed that smokers had a significantly increased risk of aseptic loosening, deep infection and revision compared with non-smokers. There was no difference in the length of hospital stay or in the risk of dislocation. Cohort studies can be prospective or retrospective.

6.9   Interventional Studies

Interventional studies is another name for clinical trials. They are very similar to prospective cohort studies, with subjects being followed prospectively after the initiation of the investigation. The important difference is that some form of intervention is introduced by researchers that has the potential to alter the occurrence or course of the disease or condition under investigation. These studies are usually viewed as the ideal type of study, providing greater evidence of causal inference than observational investigations, largely because of their prospective nature and the ability of researchers to randomise patients to receive or not receive the intervention.

Two recent examples of randomised controlled interventional studies in orthopaedic trauma are those of d'Heurle et al. [15] and Prestmo et al. [16]. d'Heurle et al. [15] undertook a prospective randomised trial of locked and non-locked plates for the treatment of high-energy distal tibial fractures and showed no difference in the results. This type of study is important as locking plates have been sold with considerable enthusiasm, and it is important for orthopaedic surgeons to know whether these more expensive implants are any better than the previous cheaper ones.

Prestmo et al. [16] studied geriatric care for patients with hip fractures. They randomly assigned home dwelling patients with hip fractures who were ≥70 years of age and were able to walk 10 m before their fractures to either comprehensive geriatric care or standard orthopaedic care. They showed that immediate admission of these patients to a comprehensive geriatric unit in a dedicated ward improved mobility at 4 months compared with the usual orthopaedic care. They concluded that the treatment of older patients with hip fractures should be organised as orthogeriatric care. This type of study is very important in that it will determine how geriatric patients with fractures should be treated in the future.

6.10   Methodological Problems

A simple review of the types of study that can be undertaken tends to obscure the complexity associated with undertaking good-quality epidemiological studies. It is often difficult to collect and analyse data. Cummings et al. [17] identified several key areas of consideration, and these are listed in Table 6.4.

Table 6.4 Important areas of methodology to consider when designing an epidemiological study

Numerator problems
The definition, classification, categorisation and ascertainment of fractures
Denominator problems
Matching numerators to denominators and selecting the appropriate denominator
Causation
Identifying and categorising the many and varied causes and mechanisms of injury
Multiplicity
The history of multiple events. Multiple fractures may occur in one patient or there may be more than one fracture during the period of study

6.11   Numerator Problems

In many medical conditions, it is relatively simple to collect data and process it. Any condition which will always present to a specialist should be relatively straightforward to analyse epidemiologically. However, this is not the case with all medical diseases or conditions. Orthopaedic trauma is a good example of this problem, and the orthopaedic literature is full of examples of imperfect collection of data regarding the type of fracture that has been seen. This is particularly problematic in descriptive studies and cross-sectional surveys.

Empirically one would think that the collection of data regarding fractures would be straightforward. One would simply go to the hospital where all the fractures are seen and assess their prevalence and incidence. However, fracture ascertainment, or the identification of fractures correctly using the available investigations, may be remarkably difficult. In many countries fractures are diagnosed and treated in different types of institution with severe trauma being treated in level 1 trauma centres, or their equivalent, while less severe trauma is treated in community hospitals or by surgeons in private practice. Thus few hospitals see the complete range of orthopaedic trauma, and, as there is usually little communication between hospitals, it is often difficult to accurately assess the prevalence and incidence of fractures.

The other problem is the experience of the doctor, or paramedical professional, who diagnoses the fractures. Some fractures are very difficult to diagnose. It is unlikely that an open femoral diaphyseal fracture will be misdiagnosed, but inexperienced medical professionals may find it difficult to diagnosis fractures of the hand, wrist and foot. Increasingly, in some countries, people with minor fractures are being assessed in minor injuries clinics, increasingly staffed by nonmedical clinicians, where a diagnosis may be arrived at with or without the use of radiography. This has the potential to lead to incorrect epidemiological results.

A recent analysis of the ability of medical and nonmedical emergency department staff to diagnose fractures showed that of 7449 fractures reviewed in the emergency department of a large hospital, an incorrect diagnosis was made in 22% of the cases [18]. Further analysis showed that junior doctors and nurses misdiagnosed 23.6% of fractures, and even senior emergency department medical staff

Table 6.5 A comparison of the incidence of fractures from different studies using different methodologies

	Study years	Country	Incidence (n/10⁵/year)		
			Overall	Male	Female
Donaldson et al. [19]	1980–82	UK	9.1	10	8.1
Johansen et al. [21]	1994–95	UK	21.1	23.5	18.8
Court-Brown and Caesar [23]	2000	UK	12.6	13.6	11.6
Rennie et al. [22]					
Donaldson et al. [20]	2002–4	UK	36.0	41.0	31.0
Sahlin [24]	1985–6	Norway	22.8	22.9	21.3
Fife and Barancik [25]	1977	USA	21.0	26.0	16.0

All studies include children and adults

misdiagnosed 17.1% of fractures. This illustrates the importance of referring trauma, however, apparently minor, to an experienced trauma surgeon if accurate epidemiological information is to be obtained.

Because of the difficulty of accurately assessing fracture epidemiology, different methods have been used in the past, with varying results. Table 6.5 gives the incidences of fractures in four studies in the United Kingdom [19–23], one in Norway [24] and one in the USA [25]. All the studies include both children and adults, and one would expect the results to be very similar. The average life expectancy and degree of deprivation is similar in the three countries, and it is highly unlikely that the overall epidemiology of fractures differs very much. However, different methodologies have been used, and we believe that this accounts for the wide variation in results that is shown in Table 6.5.

Donaldson et al. in their early study [19] examined a geographically well-defined population in England and recorded both in-patient and out-patient fractures. They thought that they might have missed some toe fractures and some spinal fractures, but they felt that they had missed relatively few injuries. Similar methodology was employed by Court-Brown and Caesar [23] and by Rennie et al. [22] in Scotland in 2000. Court-Brown and Caesar collected and analysed adult fractures, while Rennie and her co-workers collected the paediatric data during the same period. Their results have been combined to allow comparison with the results of Donaldson et al. [19]. Table 6.5 shows that the results of the two studies are similar, and it is likely that the slight differences are associated with the 20-year gap between the two studies.

However, the other studies in Table 6.5 give quite different results. The studies by Johansen et al. in Wales [21], Sahlin in Norway [24] and Fife and Barancik in the USA [25] all recorded similar fracture incidences. The methodology in these different studies was similar, with the diagnosis of the different fracture types being taken from the records of the local emergency departments. Many of the patients would have been reviewed by junior doctors or paramedical staff and would not have seen an experienced orthopaedic surgeon. This is in contrast to the Scottish studies where all diagnoses were made by orthopaedic surgeons. This is particularly likely to result in an incorrect estimate of fracture incidence in areas of the body where soft tissue injuries are common such as the hand, wrist, foot and ankle. This is illustrated by comparing the incidence of fractures in the forearm, wrist and hand in the Welsh study with the Scottish study. The relative incidences were 9.2/1000/year and 6.1/1000/year. Similar discrepancies were seen in ankle and foot fractures but not in femoral diaphyseal fractures where the incidences were 1.6/1000/year in Wales and 1.4/1000/year in Scotland. Aitken et al. [18] also showed that emergency department staff significantly misdiagnosed and overestimated the number of certain upper limb fractures (clavicle, proximal humerus, distal humerus, proximal radius, ulnar diaphysis, distal radius, carpus, metacarpus and fingers) and lower limb fractures (proximal tibia, talus, calcaneus, mid-foot, metatarsus and toes).

A third type of methodological analysis that has been employed is simply to ask patients to complete a questionnaire as to whether they have had a fracture in a given period. Table 6.5 shows that the second study by Donaldson et al. [20], which used this methodology, recorded a fracture incidence of $36/10^5$/year which is highly unlikely. It should be borne in mind that many patients are told that continuing pain may be related to an undiagnosed fracture by physiotherapists, osteopaths, other paramedical personnel and even friends and acquaintances.

In recent years epidemiological analyses have been undertaken using large databases which are often compiled by government agencies. The implication is that the size of the database improves the quality of the research. However, it is important to remember that even in large databases, the quality of the data is still affected by the skill with which the underlying medical condition is diagnosed. A good example of the problems endemic in some databases is the General Practice Research Database, now known as the Clinical Practice Research Datalink. This is widely used in the United Kingdom. The data are taken from general practices run by family physicians, but in conditions which are diagnosed in hospital, they simply store the diagnoses which are given to them. Thus the same problems apply as in the emergency department of the hospital. The database will contain many diagnoses made by non-experts. This is very likely to apply to many large databases throughout the world.

The other problem with large databases is knowing how complete they are. Some databases compiled in countries with extensive private practice may not be very complete. There is debate as to what constitutes a satisfactory database. Few have been analysed to any significant extent, but in a country with a reputation for efficiency and expertise, namely Denmark, the Danish Fracture Database was assessed as being 83% complete [26], and it was felt that surgery-related data were valid in 89–99% of cases. This probably represents a very successful database.

A recent example of the use of a large database to produce a significant conclusion is that of Nordström et al. [27]. They used the Swedish National Patient Register which covers all in-patient care provided in Sweden since 1987. They established that 116,111 patients aged ≥50 years had a primary hip fractures between 2006 and 2012. Using this large database, they were able to show that for patients who had a length of stay in hospital of ≤10 days, each 1 day reduction in length of stay increased the odds of death within 30 days of discharge by 8% in 2006 and 16% in 2012. In patients admitted for ≥11 days, reduction of length of stay was not associated with increased mortality. In many countries there have been attempts to discharge elderly patients earlier after hip fracture to free beds for other patients to use. The analysis of this very large database suggests that this may well not be in the patient's best interest!

The variability of databases was examined in a recent study of the association of benzodiazepines with proximal femoral and femoral diaphyseal fractures [28]. Three primary care databases were used from Spain, the United Kingdom and Holland. The authors pointed out that benzodiazepines increased the risk of fracture but that there were discrepancies between the databases. It is therefore important that anyone proposing to undertake an epidemiological study from any size of database be aware of who collected the data and how it was collected. It should be remembered that such databases are simply collected and used because it is relatively easy to use them. They may not be accurate.

It does seem likely that the use of large databases will increase, and it is probable that the databases will be more accurate and more sophisticated in the future. In a recent study Pugely et al. [29] analysed the large databases, available in the USA, which can be used for epidemiological studies. As an example they pointed out that Medicare is the largest and most complete administrative claims database for patients ≥65 years of age and that by 2012 there were >45 million people enrolled in Medicare. However they also pointed out that Medicare data have distinct disadvantages. The data set does not apply to the younger non-Medicare population, and the data are difficult to access and manipulate. It is also very expensive. The other problem is the accuracy of the coding system. They pointed out that there were significant inaccuracies associated with the ICD-9 coding system and that the ICD-10 coding system would be better. It is difficult to know how accurate these databases will be in the future, but there are likely to be inherent coding inaccuracies in particular, and we must hope that the sheer numbers of people in each of these large databases compensates for any inaccuracies that persist.

6.12 The Use of Subjective Numerator Criteria

It is relatively straightforward to analyse the epidemiology of fractures in terms of the bone that is involved and the location of the fracture within the bone, but to undertake a more in-depth analysis requires the use of classification systems that describe fracture morphology. Aitken et al. [30] pointed out that there are many classifications, but there is often considerable inter- and intra-observer error associated with their use. This may be minimised by having one surgeon classify all fractures, but this is frequently impractical, and with studies relying on inexperienced doctors and paramedical personnel to diagnose fractures, there will be a considerable error rate if anything more than a basic fracture classification system is used to define fractures. This problem was well illustrated by Siebenrock and Gerber [31] who analysed the Neer and AO classification systems for proximal humeral fractures. They found that neither system was sufficiently reproducible to allow meaningful comparison of similarly classified fractures in different studies.

6.13   Denominator Problems

Just as selecting the correct numerator is essential for undertaking good epidemiological studies, it is also important to select the correct denominator. It is not unusual for surgeons to assume that whatever range of fractures is seen in their hospital represents the whole community because they have not appreciated that the hospital only sees a proportion of the people in the community.

Correlational studies and cross-sectional studies require the use of a definite population, and in studies of fracture epidemiology, this is usually the geographical catchment area of the healthcare facilities used to capture the numerator database. However, it can be extremely difficult to define the correct catchment area if there is more than one hospital admitting a particular disease or condition in an area. The ideal situation is to have only one hospital responsible for a particular condition and to have no private medical practitioners involved in the treatment of the condition. If this is not the case, accurate data regarding the numerator and denominator are difficult to obtain. However this ideal situation is rare, and it is common for children and adults to be treated in different hospitals and for spinal fractures and complex hand injuries to be treated by neurosurgeons and plastic surgeons, meaning that it is difficult to obtain numerator data and denominator data with any accuracy. To undertake accurate studies, a carefully defined catchment area must be examined and specific data obtained for all patients in that area who present with the disease or condition under review. One useful technique is to use postal codes or zip codes and analyse the condition under review in these areas, but one must remember that the numerator information may still be deficient.

One example of the problems associated with the use of incorrect denominator information can be seen by examining the epidemiology of ankle fractures. These are the fourth most common fracture to present to orthopaedic surgeons with an incidence of $137.7/10^5$/year in the recent Edinburgh study of all in-patient and out-patient fractures in a defined population. Overall 1% of the ankle fractures were open [4]. A study entitled *Epidemiology of ankle fractures in Sweden between 1987 and 2004* [32] examined 91,140 ankle fractures but only analysed in-patients. The incidence was $71/10^5$/year, and 3% of the fractures were open. In a second study entitled *Epidemiology of foot and ankle fractures in the United States: An analysis of the National Trauma Data Bank (2007 to 2011)* [33], the authors did not state an incidence, but 17.9% of their ankle fractures were open. In the first paper [32] the authors recognised that they had not examined out-patients, and in the second paper [33] the authors stated that the data were collected from major trauma centres and that fracture identification depended on the quality of coding. However the titles of the papers imply that their results apply to the overall population. The differences in the incidence of ankle fractures and in the prevalence of open fractures highlight the importance of using a correct denominator and understanding exactly what the results mean.

6.14 Other Factors

There are a number of other factors that surgeons need to take into consideration. Firstly, is the database used for analysis representative of the whole population? Two examples of this type of problem are the use of large databases that do not cover the whole population and the analysis of in-patient fractures only. Clearly if one is simply wanting to know about the epidemiology of a particular proportion of the population, these methodologies are satisfactory, but they cannot be extended to the whole population as shown above with the epidemiology of ankle fractures. Another example of nonrepresentative methodology is the use of insurance databases. These cannot cover the complete population as a proportion will be uninsured. Brinker and O'Connor [34] examined the incidence of fractures in a large privately insured cohort of patients. The average age of the males was 29 years, and the average age of the females was 28.7 years. Thus the epidemiology that was examined would only represent a younger population. Bradly and Harrison [35] examined in-patients in Australia to produce information about fracture epidemiology. However, as 55–60% of fractures are seen on an out-patient basis in most healthcare systems, the information obtained from this type of study is limited and can only be applied to less than half of the fracture population.

6.15 Causation

Aitken et al. [30] pointed out that many patient-related and environmental factors contribute to the occurrence of a fracture and knowledge of this multifactorial aetiology may be necessary to define the epidemiology of a particular fracture or patient group. For example, when examining road traffic accidents as a cause of injury, researchers must allow for potential differences in exposure between subsections of the population studied. Certain patient groups, such as the elderly, may be less likely to hold a drivers licence, or drive a vehicle, putting them at inherently lower risk of sustaining injury from this cause. The same argument applies to the incidence of fractures in sports injuries. Researchers must appreciate the differing levels of sports participation, and therefore risk exposure, between groups.

6.16 Multiplicity

Surgeons should remember that when they are undertaking an epidemiological study of fractures or other medical conditions, that one patient can sustain several fractures at the same time or the patient may suffer fractures on separate occasions within the period of study. When this happens the assumption that events are statistically independent may not be correct and can complicate the analysis of the data.

Researchers need to be aware of these problems. They must decide on how the data for multiple events will be treated prior to statistical analysis and record this information in the methods section of the related manuscript.

6.17   Measures of Occurrence and Association in Epidemiological Studies

We will present the basic measures of occurrence and association commonly used in orthopaedic epidemiological studies. Epidemiologists use a wide variety of measures, and if further information is required, a specialist epidemiological text [1] should be consulted.

6.18   Occurrence

It is essential to be able to quantify the occurrence of a disease or medical condition in any epidemiological study, with the exception perhaps of case reports or case series. The simplest measure is an assessment of the number of affected individuals. In the previously quoted study by Nordström et al. [27], the simple fact that there were 116,111 hip fractures in a 7-year period in Sweden may help to determine the allocation of hospital and community resources. However, to investigate the distribution and causes of injury and disease, it is necessary to know the size of the population and the time period during which data were collected.

The most commonly used measures of the occurrence of a disease or a medical condition are prevalence and cumulative incidence. These are defined in Table 6.6.

Prevalence is the proportion of the population under scrutiny found to have a disease or a medical condition. Table 6.6 shows that it is calculated by comparing the number of people or cases found to have the condition with the total number of people or cases examined and is usually expressed as a percentage. Point prevalence is the proportion of a population that has the condition at a specific point in time. Period prevalence is the proportion of a population that has the condition at some time during the given period and includes people who already have the condition at the start of the study period. Lifetime prevalence is the proportion of a population that experienced the condition at some point in their life. As an example, in the study of fractures in Edinburgh in 2010/2011 [4] which is illustrated in Table 6.3, there were 1221 distal radial fractures identified in adults (≥16 years of age) during the 1-year study period. Given that the total number of fractures identified was 6996, the prevalence of distal radius fractures was 17.5% within the fracture patient group. Prevalence measures are particularly useful for determining resources. Thus if one knows that 17.5% of all fractures involve the distal radius, it is sensible to provide sufficiently appropriate staff and resources to treat this particular condition.

Cumulative incidence, which is usually referred to in medical studies simply as incidence, quantifies the number of newly occurring cases of a disease or condition in the population at risk over a specific time period (Table 6.6). It is

Table 6.6 Measures of occurrence and association

Prevalence
Number of cases of disease or medical condition
divided by
Number of cases studied
Cumulative incidence
Number of new cases of disease in a specific period
divided by
Total population at risk at the beginning of the study
Incidence density
Number of new cases of disease during a specific time period
divided by
Number of person-years of observation
Adjusted rate
Total number of cases of disease in a subgroup of the population
divided by
Number of individuals in that subgroup in a specific time period
Risk ratio
Incidence in exposed group of patients
divided by
Incidence in non-exposed group of patients
Odds ratio
Number of exposed cases × number of unexposed non-cases
divided by
Number of exposed non-cases × number of unexposed cases

particularly important when measuring incidence that the denominator is correct. The 1221 distal radius fractures in 2010/2011 in Edinburgh occurred in a population of 517,512 adults, giving an incidence of 235.9/100,000 population per year. This is conventionally expressed $235.9/10^5$/year [5]. This type of incidence measurement requires that the entire population has been followed up for a specific time interval, and the population number at the *beginning* of the study period is used as the denominator for calculation. However, this is not always the case, and it may be that the time of admission to the study is variable or the follow-up period varies.

Under these circumstances one can use incidence *density*, often known as incidence *rate*, rather than the cumulative incidence (Table 6.6). The main difference here is that the calculation takes account of the changing size of the population studied, and mean population size or 'summed person-years' is used as the denominator. In the case of Edinburgh distal radius fractures, there were 1221 per 517,512 person-years in 2010/2011. Hypothetically, if the report had found 2360 cases in a further 2-year study period (where the local population was found to be 520,000 in the first year, then 525,000 in the second), the incidence rate would be calculated, thus:

$$(1221 + 2360)\,\text{fractures}/(517{,}512 + 520{,}000 + 525{,}000)\,\text{person.years}$$
$$= 3581/1{,}562{,}512\,\text{person.years} = 0.002291/\text{one person.year}$$
$$= 229.1/10^5\,\text{person.years}.$$

The incidence rate can be used to determine an individual's risk of developing the disease or condition during a specified period of time. It should be noted that 'cumulative incidence' is equal to 'incidence rate' if the specified study period is 1 year.

6.19   Adjusted Rates

The occurrence of disease over time (Table 6.6) can be calculated for an entire population, this being known as the crude rate (e.g. incidence or incidence rate). Alternatively, the crude rate can be refined to reflect the influence of a particular factor within the population, e.g. patient age or gender, referred to as the age-adjusted or gender-specific rate, accordingly. The crude rate, much like the incidence, is obtained by dividing the total number of new cases by the number in that population in a specific time period. Continuing the example from above, the crude rate of distal radius fractures in adults in Edinburgh in 2010/2011 over the 1-year period was $235.9/10^5$/year. If one was keen to learn the influence of patient age on distal radius fracture incidence, then the age-adjusted rates provide more information. Comparing the 20–29-year-old population and the 70–79-year-old population, the appropriate number of fractures incurred by each age group is divided by the total number of people in these groups. The corresponding figures are 114/59,279 and 191/24,998 giving age-adjusted rates of $192.3/10^5$/year and $764.1/10^5$/year, respectively, and confirming that patient age has an influence on the occurrence of these injuries.

Epidemiologists also use adjusted rates to compensate for population variables, such as the changing size and demographics of the population over time, as these factors will contribute to the frequency with which a disease or medical condition is encountered. The incidence of distal radius fractures in adults in Edinburgh was $235.9/10^5$/year in a population numbering 517,512 adults. In 2000 there were 1009 fractures in the same population area with a population size of 508,936, giving an incidence of $198.3/10^5$/year. The increase in absolute numbers of distal radius fractures is not simply a reflection of the increasing size of the population, as the fracture incidence already controls for population size. The difference could conceivably result from a change in population demographics, such an increase in the proportion of older individuals, females or socioeconomically deprived groups. The calculation of rates, appropriately adjusted for these variables, would provide investigators with more meaningful information.

6.20   Measures of Association

In epidemiological research the calculation of the frequencies of diseases or medical conditions is the basis for the comparison of populations which allows the identification of the causes of disease. To facilitate comparison, the two frequencies being compared can be combined into a single parameter that estimates the association between an exposure to the risk of developing the disease or condition. The two commonest ratios that are used to define this association are the risk ratio and odds ratios (Table 6.6).

6.21 Risk Ratio

Risk ratio is the ratio of the probability of an event occurring in a particular 'at risk' or 'exposed' group of people, to the probability of the same event occurring in the unexposed group. As an example, this kind of calculation can highlight the influence of age and gender on the risk of fracture in a given population. However, as with other epidemiological calculations, it is vital that the denominator be correct.

An example is the risk of 80–89-year-old females sustaining a non-spinal fracture in a given year. In the 2010/2011 study in Edinburgh, there were 723 fractures in females aged 80–89 years and 6065 fractures in the remaining adult population. The respective incidences for the two groups are $4712.9/10^5$/year and $1117.6/10^5$/year, giving a risk ratio of 4.2. It is of interest that the risk ratio for an 80–89-year-old female sustaining a proximal femoral fracture when compared with the rest of the community was 19.1!

A relative risk of 1.0 indicates that the incidence rates of a disease or a condition in a particular group is the same as for the rest of the population. A value >1.0 indicates a positive association, and the ratio of 4.2 means that 80–89-year-old females are 320% (i.e. 4.2 minus the null value of 1.0) more likely to develop a fracture.

6.22 Odds Ratio

The odds ratio quantifies how strongly the presence or absence of a causative factor or variable is associated with the presence or absence of a certain disease or outcome in a given population. The risk ratio is the ratio of the probability, whereas odds ratio is the ratio of the odds. The calculation of odds ratio is explained in Table 6.6.

An example of this is an estimation of how useful reaming is in achieving union in closed tibial diaphyseal fractures [36]. This has been of interest to orthopaedic surgeons for about 20 years, and if an odds ratio had been calculated from the early papers published on this subject, it is possible that the argument would have been settled already! Six early papers [37–42] examined the role of nailing in the management of closed tibial diaphyseal fractures and quoted the numbers of fractures that united with and without reaming. There were 141 fractures out of 145 fractures that united with reaming and 146 fractures out of 173 that united without reaming. The odds ratio of reamed nailing resulting in union compared with unreamed nailing resulting in union is 141/4 divided by 146/27 or (141 × 27) / (4 × 146), i.e. 6.5. It can be seen that reaming increases the odds of achieving union in closed tibial diaphyseal fractures by a factor of greater than six times. The literature indicates that risk ratios are better understood by clinicians than odds ratios. It is also the case that odds ratios can overestimate the differences between treated groups if the trial has a high event rate.

Table 6.7 Guidelines to facilitate undertaking an epidemiological study

1. Has the correct epidemiological study been used?
2. Has the correct numerator been used? Do you know who diagnosed the condition being studied and how the information was recorded? Are all the parameters being studied properly defined?
3. Has the correct denominator been used? Has the correct population been studied? Are you extrapolating the denominator to cover an inappropriate population?
4. Have all the potential causes of the disease or condition been examined?
5. Are there multiple events that may alter the epidemiological analysis?

6.23 Conclusions

Epidemiological studies are very important in medicine, whether they be case reports that draw attention to a particular disease or treatment method for future consideration or randomised controlled interventional studies that remain the gold standard for testing treatments or investigating factors that might cause disease. They are usually straightforward to undertake, but problems with obtaining the correct numerator and denominator are not uncommon. Surgeons should be aware of the accuracy with which the diagnosis of the disease or medical condition is being made and the accuracy with which the information is being recorded. The use of large databases does not negate this problem of data acquisition.

The denominator is equally important. Not infrequently surgeons assume that what they see in their institution reflects the whole community. This is often incorrect. The population that they study must reflect the population that they wish to investigate, and they must also be aware of the size of the population that is being treated for a particular disease or medical condition. A summary of the basic requirements for an epidemiological study are given in Table 6.7.

References

1. Hennekens CH, Buring J, Mayrent SL, editors. Epidemiology in medicine. Philadelphia: Lippincott Williams and Wilkins; 1987.
2. Doll R, Hill AB. Smoking and carcinoma of the lung: preliminary report. BMJ. 1950;2(4682):739–48.
3. Stimson LA. A practical treatise on fractures and dislocations. 4th ed. New York: Lea Brothers & Co; 1905.
4. Court-Brown CM. The epidemiology of fractures and dislocations. In: Court-Brown CM, Heckman JD, McQueen MM, Ricci WM, Tornetta P, editors. Rockwood and Green's fractures in adults. 8th ed. Philadelphia: Wolters Kluwer; 2015.
5. Court-Brown CM, Aitken SA, Duckworth AD, Clement ND, McQueen MM. The relationship between social deprivation and the incidence of adult fractures. J Bone Joint Surg Am. 2013;70-A:74–9.
6. Moura CS, Abrahamowicz M, Beauchamp ME, Lacaille D, Wang Y, Boire G, Fortin PR, Bessette L, Bombardier C, Widdifield J, Hanly JG, Feldman D, Maksymowych W, Peschken C, Barnabe C, Edworthy S, Bernatsky S, CAN-AIM. Early medication use in new-onset rhenmatoid arthritis may delay joint replacement: results of a large population-based study. Arthritis Res Ther. 2015;17:197. https://doi.org/10.1186/s 13075-015-0713-3.

7. Caban-Martinez AJ, Courtney TK, Chang WR, Lombardi DA, Huang YH, Brennan MJ, Perry MJ, Katz JN, Christiani DC, Verma SK. Leisure-time physical activity, falls and fall injuries in middle-aged adults. Am J Prev Med. 2015;49(6):888–901. https://doi.org/10.1016/j.amepre.2015.05.022.
8. Song KS, Lee SW. Subtrochanteric femur fracture after removal of screws for femoral neck fracture in a child. Am J Orthop. 2015;44:40–2.
9. Paraliticci G, Rodríguez-Quintana R, Dávilla A, Otero-López A. Atraumatic bilateral femoral neck fractures in a premenopausal female with hypovitaminosis D. Bol Assoc Med PR. 2015;107:51–4.
10. Centers for Disease Control. Pneumocystis pneumonia-Los Angeles. MMWR. 1981;30:250.
11. Braun KF, Pohlig F, Lenze U, Netter C, Hadjamu M, Rechl H, von Eisenhart-Rothe R. Insufficiency fractures after irradiation therapy – case series. MMW Fortschr Med. 2015; 157(Suppl 5):1–4.
12. Sarosiek S, Sehlin DC, Connors LH, Spencer B, Murakami A, O'Hare C, Sanchorawala V. Vertebral compression fractures as the initial presentation of AL amyloidosis: case series and review of the literature. Amyloid. 2015;24:1–7.
13. Bishop J, Agel J, Dunbar R. Predictive factors for knee stiffness after periarticular fracture: a case-control study. J Bone Joint Surg. 2012;94-A:1833–8.
14. Teng S, Yi C, Krettek C, Jagodzinski M. Smoking and risk of prosthesis-related complications after total hip arthroplasty: a meta-analysis of cohort studies. PLoS One. 2015;10(4):e0125294.
15. d'Heurle A, Kazemi N, Connelly C, Wyrick JD, Archdeacon MT, Le TT. Prospective randomized comparison of locked plates versus nonlocked plates for the treatment of high-energy pilon fractures. J Orthop Trauma. 2015;29:420–3.
16. Prestmo A, Hagen G, Sletvold O, Helbostad JL, Thingstad P, Taraldsen K, Lydersen S, Halsteinli V, Saltnes T, Lamb SE, Johnsen LG, Saltvedt I. Comprehensive geriatric care for patients with hip fractures: a prospective, randomised, controlled trial. Lancet. 2015;385(9978):1623–33.
17. Cummings P, Koepsell TD, Mueller BA. Methodological challenges in injury epidemiology and injury prevention research. Annu Rev. Public Health. 1995;16:381–400.
18. Aitken SA, Rodrigues MA, Duckworth AD, Clement ND, McQueen MM, Court-Brown CM. Determining the incidence of adult fractures: how accurate are emergency department data? Epidemiol Res Int. 2012;2012:837928. https://doi.org/10.1155/2012/837928.
19. Donaldson LJ, Cook A, Thomson RG. Incidence of fractures in a geographically defined population. J Epidemiol Community Health. 1990;44:241–5.
20. Donaldson LJ, Reckless IP, Scholes S, Mindell JS, Shelton NJ. The epidemiology of fractures in England. J Epidemiol Community Health. 2008;62:174–80.
21. Johansen A, Evans RJ, Stone MD, Stone MD, Richmond PW, Lo SV, Woodhouse KW. Fracture incidence in England and Wales: a study based on the population of Cardiff. Injury. 1997;28:655–60.
22. Rennie L, Court-Brown CM, Mok JY, Beattie TF. The epidemiology of fractures in children. Injury. 2007;38:913–22.
23. Court-Brown CM, Caesar B. Epidemiology of adult fractures. A review. Injury. 2006;30:691–7.
24. Sahlin Y. Occurrence of fractures in a defined population: a 1-year study. Injury. 1990;21:158–60.
25. Fife D, Barancik J. Norteastern Ohio trauma study III: incidence of fractures. Ann Emerg Med. 1985;14:244–8.
26. Gromov K, Fristed JV, Brix M, Troelsen A. Completeness and data validity for the Danish fracture database. Dan Med J. 2013;60:A4712.
27. Nordström P, Gustafson Y, Michaëlsson K, Nordström A. Length of hospital stay after hip fracture and short term risk of death after discharge: a total cohort study in Sweden. BMJ. 2015;350:h696. https://doi.org/10.1136/bmj.h696.
28. Requena G, Huerta C, Gardarsdottir H, Logie J, González-González R, Abbing-Karahagopian V, Miret M, Schneider C, Souverein PC, Webb D, Afonso A, Boudiaf N, Martin E, Oliva B, Alvarez A, De Groot MC, Bate A, Johansson S, Schlienger R, Reynolds R, Klungel OH, de Abajo FJ. Hip/femur fractures associated with the use of benzodiazepines (anxiolytics, hypnotics and related drugs): a methodological approach to assess consistencies across databases from the PROJECT-EU project. Pharmacoepidemiol Drug Saf. 2015;25(Suppl 1):66–78. https://doi.org/10.1002/pds.3816.

29. Pugely AJ, Martin CT, Harwood J, Ong KL, Bozic KJ, Callaghan JJ. Database and regis-
    try research in orthopaedic surgery. Part 1: claims-based data. J Bone Joint Surg Am.
    2015;97:1278–87.
30. Aitken SA, Hutchison JD, McQueen MM, Court-Brown CM. The importance of epidemio-
    logical fracture data. Bone Joint J. 2014;96-B:863–7.
31. Siebenrock KA, Gerber C. The reproducibility of classification of fractures of the proximal
    end of the humerus. J Bone Joint Surg Am. 1993;75-A:1751–5.
32. Thur CK, Edgren G, Jansson K-Å, Wretenberg P. Epidemiology of adult ankle fractures in
    Sweden between 1987 and 2004. Acta Orthop. 2012;83:276–81.
33. Shibuya N, Davis ML, Jupiter DC. Epidemiology of foot and ankle fractures in the United
    States: an analysis of the national trauma data bank (2007 to 2011). J Foot Ankle Surg.
    2014;53:606–8.
34. Brinker MR, O'Connor DP. The incidence of fractures and dislocations referred for orthopae-
    dic services in a capitated population. J Bone Joint Surg Am. 2004;86-A:291–7.
35. Bradley C, Harrison J. Descriptive epidemiology of traumatic fractures in Australia. Injury
    search and statistics. Series Number 17. Adelaide AIHW (AIHW cat no INJ-CAT 57); 2004.
36. Court-Brown CM. Fractures of the tibia and fibula. In: Bucholz RW, Heckman JD, editors.
    Rockwood and Green's fractures in adults. 5th ed. Philadelphia: Lippincott Williams and
    Wilkins; 2001.
37. Court-Brown CM, Will E, Christie J, McQueen MM. Reamed or unreamed nailing for closed
    tibial fractures. J Bone Joint Surg (Br). 1996;78-B:580–3.
38. Blachut PA, O'Brien PJ, Meek RN, Broekhuyse HM. Interlocking intramedullary nailing with
    and without reaming for the treatment of closed fractures of the tibial shaft. J Bone Joint Surg
    Am. 1997;79-A:640–6.
39. Bone LB, Sucato D, Stegemann PM, Rohrbacher BJ. Displaced isolated fractures of
    the tibial shaft treated with either a cast or intramedullary nailing. J Bone Joint Surg Am.
    1997;79-A:1336–41.
40. Gregory P, Sanders R. Treatment of closed, unstable tibial shaft fractures with unreamed inter-
    locking nails. Clin Orthop. 1995;315:48–55.
41. Krettek C, Schandelmaier P, Tscherne H. Non-reamed interlocking nailing of closed tibial
    fractures with severe soft tissue injury. Clin Orthop. 1995;315:34–47.
42. Riemer BL, DiChristina DG, Cooper A, Sagiv S, Butterfield SL, Burke CJ, Lucke JF, Schlosser
    JD. Nonreamed nailing of tibial diaphyseal fractures in blunt polytrauma patients. J Orthop
    Trauma. 1999;13:27–32.

Common Causes of Rejection

7

Fredric M. Pieracci

7.1 Introduction

Medical writing and publication have changed dramatically over the last century. The theatrical prose of the nineteenth and early twentieth century has given way to methodical, regimented reporting structures. One may contrast Samuel Gross's well-known description of shock in 1862 as the "rude unhinging of the machinery of life" to that of the author's recent description as "a state of tissue dysoxia in which oxygen delivery is insufficient to meet metabolic demands" [1]. Although the former is far more eloquent, it would almost certainly be more likely to be rejected by a contemporary journal.

Most of the change in medical writing style has been the result of an explosion of both information and knowledge. When little is known about a disease process, it is harder to describe, tempting the author to invoke whimsical imagery. However, such editorializing is a common deterrent to reviewers and ultimate cause of rejection. An additional reason for the change in writing style has been a refinement of the scientific method. Descriptive studies and conjecture have given way to hypothesis-driven research, which biostatistical methodology is used to either reject or accept the null hypothesis. Research that does not clearly adhere to this model is more likely to be rejected. Finally, the exponential growth of the number of researchers, as well as the ease with which information is disseminated, has overwhelmed many journals with submissions. Nearly as much time needs to be spent deciding to which journal a manuscript will be submitted as to composing the manuscript itself. Indeed, an unchanged version of a manuscript is frequently accepted by a journal after rejection from another journal with a similar impact factor, but different scope.

F.M. Pieracci
Denver Health Medical Center, University of Colorado School of Medicine,
Denver, CO, USA
e-mail: fredric.pieracci@dhha.org

© Springer International Publishing AG 2018
C. Mauffrey, M.M. Scarlat (eds.), *Medical Writing and Research Methodology for the Orthopaedic Surgeon*, https://doi.org/10.1007/978-3-319-69350-7_7

This chapter will review common causes of rejection and strategies to mitigate them.

7.2   What Are the Challenges?

- Rejection almost universally involves violation of one or more of the following five principles: novelty, relevance, scope, quality, and style.
- *Novelty*: Novelty refers to the originality of the work. The manuscript must contribute something new to the field. Such contribution(s) should be clearly highlighted in both the abstract and introduction.
- *Relevance*: Novel subject matter with no relevance to the contemporary care of the patient will not interest reviewers. Attempt to read the manuscript from the perspective of a surgeon caring for a patient with the particular disease or treatment that is discussed in the manuscript. Think critically about the purview and readership of the journal to which the work will be submitted.
- *Scope*: Scope refers to the balance between too little and too much information. The manuscript must have a clear statement of the problem, as well as an organized hypothesis. The results should present information that is relevant only to the hypothesis. Similarly, the discussion section should only draw conclusions from the results presented. Do not inundate the reviewer with too many results. Rather, select between five and ten key results to be presented in the body of the manuscript. Moreover, too little information covered up by prose is most often readily discovered and rejected by seasoned reviewers.
- *Quality*: Study design should have a reasonable chance of a positive outcome. Common study limitations, such as inadequate sample size, confounding, and attrition, should be anticipated and addressed clearly in the manuscript. Positive results should be highlighted, and negative results should be explained with respect to additional information gleaned. Routine consultation with a biostatistician is recommended.
- *Style*: Medical writing follows a particular style. Avoid editorializing, dramatic and flamboyant prose, and extraneous information. List only the facts; the manuscript should be purposefully "dry," presenting the results and then guiding the reader to the conclusions. By contrast, the title, although concise, should be both "eye catching" and intriguing. Avoid lengthy introductions and conclusions. The necessity of every sentence should be questioned.

7.3   Tips and Tricks for a Successful Submission

7.3.1   Novelty

In general, reproduction of a previously published study is unlikely to result in publication. However, there are some exceptions to this rule. For example, repeating a study using a much larger sample size, different environment of care (e.g., safety net hospital, rural hospital, etc.), different patient population (e.g., socioeconomic demographics, morbid obesity, diabetes mellitus), or different geographic location will increase the novelty of the manuscript. Such improvements upon the index research should be clearly noted within the manuscript.

Outside of these specific situations, manuscripts submitted for publication should represent novel research. As such, the introduction section should succinctly relay the story of the line of research, beginning with formation of the research question and followed by research that has been conducted to date, noting existing deficiencies in the field. This delineation will set the stage for the current line of research. Whenever possible, the author's own research should be referenced, as this both builds credibility and documents prior success with publications.

7.3.2   Relevance

Novelty must be accompanied by relevance. Important unanswered questions in the field are most often ascertained by review of the current literature, abstracts from national meetings, and recent book chapters. In general, practical clinical issues are more likely to hold a reviewer's attention than obscure minutia. Many commonly practiced techniques have been passed down based on "expert opinion" when, in fact, there are little to no data to support them. Although the author is usually convinced that the research is relevant, the reviewer may not be. Accordingly, use the introduction to articulate the problem, describing disease demographics, prevalence, and any changes in disease characteristics over time. For example, "Blunt splenic trauma is present in approximately one third of all trauma admissions. Over the last two decades, there has been a shift from operative to non-operative management of blunt splenic injury. This shift has resulted in the problem of timing of venous thromboembolism prophylaxis is such patients." If a reviewer does not believe that the work is relevant, it will be rejected, regardless of its quality.

Only the minority of publications will involve multicenter, randomized clinical trials. Rather, most manuscripts report a single center or even single surgeon's experience. Some attention toward the issue of generalizability must be given within the manuscript. Convince the reviewer that the single institution's experience applies to the generic hospital, or surgeon, who may be adopting the treatment.

Finally, choose the journal to which the work will be submitted carefully. Read the journal's mission statement and readership information on line. Peruse current issues of the journal for content and relevance to your research.

7.3.3   Scope

Reviewer's rarely hold focused attention on a manuscript for more than 15 min. Accordingly, avoid lengthy and general descriptions of the research; rather, be succinct and specific. Include only enough background to educate the reviewer so that he or she may place your research into context. Similarly, every attempt should be made to hone in on only one or two hypotheses. Additional hypotheses, subgroup analyses, and discussion lines should be minimized. Moreover, the discussion and conclusion sections should extrapolate only on the results presented. Avoid conjecture and speculation not supported by the results.

7.3.4 Quality

Quality is perhaps the most important component of a successful submission. Novel and relevant work with a reasonable scope must be both well designed and contribute something meaningful to the field. Quality research begins with sound study design. In general, case reports and case series are considered descriptive as opposed to true research. By contrast, research involves hypothesis testing utilizing a dependent and independent variable. The most commonly published study designs include case control, cohort, and clinical trial. The reader is referred to several epidemiology texts for a more detailed description of study design [2–5]. The study design and dependent and independent variables should be clearly stated in the methods section. Study feasibility is assessed by estimating both effect and sample size and cross-referencing this information against the anticipated number of study subjects. This exercise will minimize the change of a type two error (failure to reject a false null hypothesis). In general, positive results that do not achieve statistical significance are less likely to be published. If the authors are not familiar with basic biostatistical analysis, the assistance of an independent biostatistician should be sought. Most journals now retain such a consultant, and errors in statistical technique are readily identified. In short, quality refers to both rigorous study design and positive results.

7.3.5 Style

Style refers to the overall feel of the manuscript, beginning with the title. The title should be concise; in general, limit the title to less than 15 words. Furthermore, the title should be a strong summary statement of the results of the study. Consider the following two titles, "The relationship between surgical fixation of rib fractures and outcomes among a cohort of critically ill trauma patients with a diverse pattern of fractures and injuries" vs. "Surgical fixation of rib fractures reduces mortality and improves pulmonary outcomes." The first title is too long and merely alludes to an association. By contrast, the second title is both concise (11 words) and makes a positive statement about the study results. In general, these same rules apply to the remainder of the manuscript. A detailed review for grammar, punctuation, and typographical errors is essential, particularly if the manuscript is being written in a non-primary language of the authors. Editorializing, conjecture, and melodramatic prose should be avoided. Moreover, certain words are commonly misused in medical writing. For example, the word "significant" has a very specific, statistical meaning in medical writing, usually connoting a P value of less than 0.05. Avoid using this word in other contexts, such as "over the last 10 years there has been a significant change in surgeons' preferences for clavicle fixation." Finally, avoid maligning other authors in the field. Rather, limitations of previous work should be stated objectively.

The introduction should comprise five to ten sentences and "set the stage" for the current research. The first one to two sentences should be devoted to a statement of the problem and its relevance, for example, "Rib fractures are the most common chest injury in trauma patients and carry a morbidity of up to 50%." Next, describe past efforts to manage the problem (including the authors' own) and limitations. Finally, state the hypothesis of the current study and how it plans to build upon the current state of the art. The hypothesis should be clearly stated and, in general, the last sentence of the introduction, for example, "the hypothesis of the current study is that surgical fixation of rib fractures, as compared to best medical management, improves pulmonary outcomes."

The methods section similarly follows a standardized outline. The first paragraph should describe the study context, e.g., academic medical center, laboratory animals, and rural outpatients. Next, the study design and sample should be clearly stated. For example, "This was a prospective cohort study of patients with rib fractures admitted to the intensive care unit." Inclusion and exclusion criteria are clearly stated. Next, primary dependent and independent variables are delineated, followed by covariates and, finally, by statistical analysis. Avoid lengthy descriptions of additional outcomes; in general, limit the analysis to primary, secondary, and, rarely, tertiary outcomes. Whenever possible, reference methodological techniques that will be used in the manuscript. Common examples that should be referenced include validation of scores (e.g., pain scores, quality of life measurements), surgical techniques, and animal models of a particular disease process. Many organizations have put forth detailed structural regulations for the reporting of clinical trials, and the reader is encouraged to read the latest iteration of the CONSORT statement [6].

The results section should contain only results. Although this statement appears self-evident, many times sentences (or even entire paragraphs) that are more appropriate for either the methods or discussion section are presented within the results section. Consider the following sentence: "Denver Health Medical Center is a state-verified Level I trauma center." This sentence is more appropriate for the methods section. Consider next the following text, "Patients in the study arm enjoyed an average of two days fewer on the ventilator, likely due to the additional chest wall stability offered by the surgical fixation." First, the use of the word "enjoyed" is inappropriately dramatic; "incurred," "used," or "were found to have" would be more appropriate for a scientific article. Second, the notion that the difference in results may be due to an increase in chest wall stability is speculative and not supported by the results; this phrase belongs in the discussion section.

The discussion section typically begins with a restatement of the identified scope of the problem, followed by a concise summary of the results. Next, a comparison to similar articles is made, highlighting specific differences in study populations, surgical techniques, limitations, and outcomes. At least one paragraph should be devoted to enumeration of study limitations. This endeavor involves a certain amount of tact; whereas the authors should attempt to convince the reviews that they are aware of important study limitations, a "laundry list" of such limitations detracts from the manuscript's credibility. Following discussion of the limitations, a clear conclusion and recommendation should be offered, including next steps in the particular line of research.

A certain style is also required when responding to reviewer's comments. The response should begin with a cover letter thanking the journal for a detailed review of the manuscript and the opportunity to improve it. Responses should then be organized in a bullet point format, with each response preceded by its individual reviewer comment. As in the manuscript, responses should be devoid of editorializing and negative tone. With very rare exception, all reviewer comments should be incorporated into the manuscript. This task usually involves a simple modification, such as adding a sentence to the limitation paragraph of the discussion section. Disagreeing with a reviewer's comment will serve only to increase the likelihood of rejection and is discouraged. In the most extreme scenarios in which it is impossible to agree with and incorporate a reviewer's comment, this should be done politely and with ample justification.

7.4   Common Mistakes and How to Prevent Them

- *Failure to review literature prior to submission*: With hundreds of articles published monthly, the authors are encouraged to review the literature the week or even day prior to submission. Discussion and citation of current articles demonstrate knowledge within the field and increase the chances of publication.
- *Submission to the wrong journal*: Spend some time reviewing various journal's websites, paying attention to mission statement, type of work considered, and scope of readership. Peruse through current and back issues, looking for relevance to the work to be submitted.
- *Too many authors*: Manuscripts with greater than ten authors (if even allowed by the journal) are in general a red flag. Limit the authorship to less than eight, and clearly state the contributions of each of the authors at the conclusion of the manuscript.
- *Inadequate/absent cover letter*: The cover letter is the first thing that both the editor and reviewers will read. Take some time to respectfully thank the journal for considering the work, and describe the relevance to the field, as well as the readership of the journal.
- *Disparaging other's work*: It is unprofessional to disparage other researches in the manuscript. Limitations of existing research should be noted in a professional manner, as well as strengths of other's contributions to the field.
- *Poor grammar*: This issue is discussed in detail in another chapter. In general, avoid colloquialisms, slang, contractions, run-on sentences, and paragraphs with only one sentence in them. The reader is referred to Strunk's *The Elements of Style* [7].
- *Ignoring formatting guidelines*: Although this issue is generally not the purview of reviewers, those who regularly review manuscripts become accustom to that

journal's formatting. Take the time to follow the formatting guidelines methodically, including headings, word limits, figure number and quality, references, etc. Failure to follow guidelines will increase the likelihood of rejection.

- *Lack of hypothesis*: The last sentence of every introduction section should contain the study hypothesis. Manuscripts will be rejected based only on this criterion.
- *Conclusion either does not answer hypothesis or is not supported by the results*: Avoid extrapolation and speculation in the conclusion. The hypothesis sentence and first sentence of the conclusion should be mirror images.
- *Failure to involve a biostatistician*: Most journals now retain statisticians who routinely review each manuscript. Biostatisticians will provide valuable information regarding study design, sample size calculation, data analysis, and articulation of study limitations.
- *Failure to have the work proofread by a colleague*: Every manuscript benefits from another set of eyes. Have the work proofread by at least one colleague, mentor, student, spouse, or good friend. Each typographical error that is corrected adds to the clarity of the work.
- *Negative or confrontational responses to reviewer's comments*: Make every effort to address each of the reviewer's comments, even if you do not agree with them. If it is not possible to revise the work based on the reviewer's comments, give a polite and detailed explanation. Most manuscripts that advance to the revisions stage will ultimately be published; curt or unprofessional responses serve only to increase the chances of ultimate rejection.

7.5 Take-Home Message

- In most cases rejection may be anticipated by a critical analysis of the manuscript's novelty, relevance, scope, quality, and style.
- Standardized formatting of all aspects of the manuscript, discussed herein, will maximize the success of submission.
- There is no substitute for clear, hypothesis-driven study design, regardless of the study findings.
- Enlist the assistance of both proofreaders and biostatisticians liberally; rampant typographical errors alone are reason for rejection.
- Most manuscripts returned with requested revisions are ultimately accepted; take this step seriously and avoid confrontation with the reviewers.

References

1. Pieracci FM, Biffl WL, Moore EE. Current concepts in resuscitation. J Intensive Care Med. 2012;27:79–96.
2. Drummond MF. Methods for the economic evaluation of health care programmes. 2nd ed. Oxford: Oxford University Press; 1997. 305 pp.

3. Pagano M, Gauvreau K. Principles of biostatistics. 2nd ed. Pacific Grove: Duxbury; 2000.
4. Kelsey JL. Methods in observational epidemiology. Monographs in epidemiology and biosta-tistics, vol. viii. 2nd ed. New York: Oxford University Press; 1996. 432 pp.
5. Friedman LM, Furberg C, DeMets DL. Fundamentals of clinical trials, vol. xviii. 3rd ed. New York: Springer; 1998. 361 pp.
6. Moher D, Schulz KF, Altman D. The CONSORT statement: revised recommendations for improving the quality of reports of parallel-group randomized trials. JAMA. 2001;285:1987–91.
7. Strunk W, White EB. The elements of style, vol. xviii. 50th Anniversary ed. New York: Pearson Longman; 2009. 105 pp.

Tips and Tricks for Non-English Writers

8

Matthew P. Abdel and Matthieu Ollivier

8.1 Introduction

All non-native English speakers (NNESs) confront cultural differences, language barriers, and grammatical peculiarities when trying to publish their work in international peer-reviewed journals written in English [1].

Foremost, writing in English is cognitively demanding for NNESs, making the process more time-consuming. Second, the presence of linguistic errors and/or poor rhetorical style in a manuscript can negatively influence the outcome of the peer-reviewed process [2]. Finally, understanding peer-reviewed publication rules is mandatory to avoid ethical issues.

The aims of this chapter are to define the main challenges for NNESs to publish in English language journals and to propose adaptive solutions for those challenges.

8.2 What Are the Challenges?

- My English vocabulary and grammar are inadequate.
- The use of my scientific language in English is even more limited.
- I do not understand the peer-reviewed publishing rules (format, style, etc.).
- My paper was rejected. What should I do now?

M.P. Abdel (✉) • M. Ollivier
Department of Orthopedic Surgery, Mayo Clinic, Rochester, MN, USA
e-mail: abdel.matthew@mayo.edu

© Springer International Publishing AG 2018
C. Mauffrey, M.M. Scarlat (eds.), *Medical Writing and Research Methodology for the Orthopaedic Surgeon*, https://doi.org/10.1007/978-3-319-69350-7_8

8.3 Common Mistakes and How to Prevent Them

8.3.1 My English Vocabulary and Grammar Are Inadequate

Non-native English speakers who are publishing in peer-reviewed scientific journal may use electronic tools such as spell check and grammar check. However, it is essential for authors to be aware that these are simple tools, and should not be relied upon heavily as they are often inaccurate, and not designed for the nuances of scientific writing. In our opinion, software and online tools that assist with translation of manuscripts should be avoided as they often result in manuscripts that are barely legible.

To prevent such errors, a host of maneuvers can be undertaken. The most reliable method is a fundamental grasp of the English language through courses for the author(s). If this is not possible, a native English speaker may be able to review your manuscript prior to submission [3]. In addition, many institutions across the world have writing centers that may assist with the process.

There are several forms of language professionals that may assist with manuscript preparation and publication. These include authors' editors, copy editors, and proofreaders [4]. An authors' editor or a copy editor is a person who works for an author and helps him/her improve the language and presentation of a manuscript before it is submitted to a journal. The work of those editors varies widely from modifying spelling and grammatical sentences to adjusting paragraph and sentence structure.

On the other hand, a proofreader is someone who is involved in the final stages of the publishing process. A proofreader examines a manuscript for grammar, typographical, and stylistic errors, but does not check whether sentences and paragraphs convey the intended meaning.

8.3.2 The Use of My Scientific Language in English Is Even More Limited

When it comes to publishing in English language journals, the philosophical differences between languages can be even more difficult to grasp than the grammatical ones. Written English for medical purposes tends to be more concise and finite than that of other languages. For NNESs, this introduces another layer of complexity. As such, many NNESs believe that the standard introduction, methods, results, and discussion format will produce acceptable scientific articles.

8.3.2.1 What Should I Do?

First, helpful checklists are available for each type of manuscript. These include the Consolidated Standards of Reporting Trials (CONSORT) checklist for randomized clinical trials (www.consort-statement.org), the Strobe checklist for cohort studies (http://www.strobe-statement.org), or Prisma for meta-analysis and systematic reviews (http://www.prisma-statement.org). In addition, it is essential for authors to know that nearly all journals have exhaustive templates that can be located on their respective websites. These checklists and templates are powerful tools that will help to improve rhetorical language and scientific style.

Another helpful tip is to download, read, and truly study well-designed, well-executed, and well-written publications from the journal you are targeting. This can give an author great insight into successful techniques.

Finally, and maybe most importantly, manuscripts should be drafted, reviewed, and edited several times. After that, they should be circulated to coauthors and then reviewed and edited once again before any consideration to submission.

8.3.3 I Do Not Understand the Peer-Reviewed Publishing Rules

8.3.3.1 Funding
There are several important rules to understand in publishing [5]. These rules may vary based upon the journal someone submits to. Foremost, it is important to be transparent. Who funded the work? Does this have the potential to introduce any bias? Who owns the data?

8.3.3.2 Authorship
In addition, authorship, and authorship order, is essential. Who actually participated in the scientific investigation, and are they worthy of authorship? In our opinion, authorship should be determined early in the investigation with clearly defined roles. The list of authors should accurately reflect those who did the intellectual work.

8.3.3.3 Redundant Publications
Redundant publications that include the same data set are unethical and dishonest. If a paper is published in any peer-reviewed journal, it cannot be published in another journal. Abstracts and posters presented at conferences are just that, presentations. As such, they do not preclude publication.

The Committee on Publication Ethics (COPE; http://publicationethics.org) provides additional information surrounding redundant work [6].

8.3.3.4 Conflict of Interest
Conflicts of interest can come in several forms, with financial conflicts being the most obvious [5]. All involved in publishing peer-reviewed manuscripts, including editors, reviewers, and authors, have a responsibility to disclose interests that might appear to impact their ability to present or review data objectively. In addition to financial conflicts of interest, there are personal, political, intellectual, and/or religious conflicts. Of note, the existence of a conflict of interest (e.g., employment with a research funder) does not preclude someone from being listed as an author if qualified.

8.3.3.5 Plagiarism and Copyright

Journal editors and readers have a right to expect that submitted work is the authors' own [4], that it has not been plagiarized (i.e., taken from other authors without permission, if permission is required), and that copyright has not been breached (e.g., reproduced figures or tables). Most journals now have advanced software [7, 8] that is able to detect the concern for plagiarism if more than 10% of a manuscript is similar to another paper.

If there is an instance of substantive plagiarism (i.e., copying more than 25% of the published source), the redundant manuscript should be withdrawn from the publication process and actions taken to inform respective institution(s). If plagiarism is surfaced after the publication, editors should retract the paper and inform the readership on misconduct.

To avoid plagiarism, the following will help:

- Provide citations with complete reference when reporting someone else's idea.
- Paraphrase rather than copy.
- Limit copying to six consecutive words.
- Obtain permission to reproduce copyrighted elements.

8.3.4 My Paper Was Rejected. What Should I Do Now?

The distinction between "nonacceptance" and "rejection" is not clear to many authors. In fact, many authors interpret nonacceptance as a rejection. Getting a paper published is sometimes a very long road. Typically, a nonacceptance allows authors the opportunity to respond to the editor and reviewer(s) with a modified manuscript.

It is important for authors to submit to journals that are appropriate for their work. Certainly, a large burden is on the author to utilize the templates and recommendations of each journal.

8.4 Take-Home Messages

- Avoid spelling and grammatical errors by reviewing and editing your manuscripts several times before submission. A native English speaker versed in scientific writing may be able to assist if questions remain.
- Be sure to understand the rules and regulations, as well as format, of the journal you are submitting to.
- Be patient and persistent with edits from editors and reviewers. Be sure to address each and every comment from the journal.

References

1. Van Weijen D. How to overcome common obstacles to publishing in English. Res Trends. 2013;35:17–8.
2. Uzuner S. Multilingual scholars participation in core/global academic communities: a literature review. J Engl Acad Purp. 2008;7(4):250–63.
3. Ravi M. Publishing a journal in English: tips for journal editors who are non-native English speakers. Sci Editing. 2014;1(1):46–8.
4. Masic I. Plagiarism in scientific publishing. Acta Inform Med. 2012;20(4):208–13.
5. Horton R. Conflicts of interest in clinical research: opprobrium or obsession? Lancet. 1997;349:1112–3.
6. Surgery Journal Editors Group. Consensus statement on the adoption of the COPE guidelines. Am J Surg. 2010;200(1):1.
7. Graf C, Deakin L, Docking M, Jones J, Joshua S, et al. Best practice guidelines on publishing ethics: a publisher's perspective. Ann N Y Acad Sci. 2014;1334(Suppl 1):e1–e23.
8. Gipp B. Citation-based plagiarism detection: detecting disguised and cross-language plagiarism using citation pattern analysis. Berkeley: Springer Vieweg; 2014. p. 10. ISBN 978-3-658-06393-1.

Impact Factor and Altmetrics: What Is the Future?

Costas Papakostidis and Peter V. Giannoudis

9.1 Introduction

The huge volume of academic literature that has been produced so far requires the use of specific tools for ascertaining quality, importance, and relevance. Traditionally, peer review, citation counting, and journal impact factor (JIF) have been used to assess the quality of scholarly work and filter out the most important and relevant scholarly material. Peer review, however, is a slow and conventional process that fails, in most instances, to filter out the volume of scholarly work (as most authors eventually succeed in publishing their work somewhere), while citation counting is even slower than peer review and insufficient to isolate influential work (which may remain uncited). The JIF is a measure reflecting the average number of citations received per paper published in a certain journal during the two preceding years [1]. While impact factor is frequently used as a measure of the relative importance of a journal within its field, it is not appropriate for assessing the quality of individual articles. Usually, a small number of a journal's articles contribute to the journal's IF, while the article under consideration may only have a very limited number of citations. In addition, editorial policy sometimes require that authors of submitted articles cite other articles that appear in the journal or commissions review articles, which generally tend to receive more citations. For these reasons a movement against inappropriate use of JIF has taken shape. A group of editors and publishers of scholarly journals met during the annual meeting of the American Society for Cell Biology (ASCB) in San Francisco, CA, on December 16, 2012, and developed a set of recommendations, referred to as the San Francisco Declaration on Research Assessment (DORA), aiming to improve the ways in which the output of scientific research is evaluated [2]. Although traditional metric tools, such as citation

C. Papakostidis • P.V. Giannoudis (✉)
Academic Department Trauma and Orthopaedic Surgery, School of Medicine, University of Leeds, Leeds, UK
e-mail: pgiannoudi@aol.com

© Springer International Publishing AG 2018
C. Mauffrey, M.M. Scarlat (eds.), *Medical Writing and Research Methodology for the Orthopaedic Surgeon*, https://doi.org/10.1007/978-3-319-69350-7_9

reference count and JIF, will remain an important component of research assessment, they steadily fail to keep pace with the continuously evolving new forms of research output and scholars' interactions with them.

9.2   What Are the Challenges that Researchers Face in the Modern Era?

• Domination of digital environment over the classical print-based world.
• New forms of scholarly outputs are gaining ground.
• A growing tendency to assess the societal impact of research.
• Poor performance of classical tools in tracking and evaluating the new forms of Web-driven research outputs as well as the impact of individual articles.
• Need for development of alternative metric tools to meet modern research requirements.

The domination of the Web as a means of communicating scientific activity has resulted in the development of new forms of scholarly output, including research datasets, posters and presentations at conferences, electronic theses, blogs, online teaching activities (such as classes, lectures), etc.

The continuously expanding volume of Web-driven academic work has set new standards for reliable evaluation and filtering of the most important and relevant scholarly material out of a huge volume of accrued scientific work. On the other hand, there has been a shift in recent years from the general assumption that research should be conducted, communicated, and evaluated only within the scientific community, toward a more open approach that tends to take into account its impact on the society. While in the past science was the core of interest of the academic community, currently, there is much concern in demonstrating its value to society [3, 4].

New metric tools have surfaced in order to measure the impact of scholarship under the currently established circumstances. While the traditionally used bibliometrics for evaluation of the impact of research have been focused on journal level (such as impact factor) or researcher level (such as h-index [5]), the newly developed metric tools concentrate on article level and on society. These alternative metric tools are referred to as altmetrics, a term coined by Jason Priem and his colleagues in 2010 to describe metric tools that focus both on individual article assessment and evaluation of the impact of alternative scholarly outputs [6]. These newly emerged metric tools are based on article level and utilize social Web for analyzing and informing scholarship, and in no case they should be considered as a surrogate to traditional metrics, but rather as a complement to them.

The article-level metrics (ALMs) include both traditional tools of impact (such as citation counts) and newer metrics like the number of times an article was downloaded. The biggest limitation of ALMs is their inability to distinguish quality within the collected feedback a scholarly output received. Altmetrics in essence represent Web-based metric tools designed to gauge the societal impact of publications and other scholarly material by using data derived from social media platforms [7, 8]. So far, a number of tools have been developed aiming at capturing and displaying these alternative metrics (altmetrics). A brief description of the most prominent of these tools is provided below:

- Altmetric. It tracks social media sites, newspapers, and magazines for any mentions of hundreds of thousands of scholarly articles. Altmetric then creates a score for each article, representing both quantitative and qualitative measure of the attention that a scholarly article has received.
- ImpactStory. It is an open-source altmetric tool that draws relevant data from a variety of social and scholarly data sources, including Facebook, Twitter, CiteULike, Delicious, PubMed, Scopus, CrossRef, ScienceSeeker, Mendeley, Wikipedia, SlideShare, etc. Altmetrics are reported in both raw numbers and percentiles compared to a sample of articles published the same year.
- Plum Analytics. They track metrics for various scholarly outputs, including journal articles, book chapters, datasets, presentations, and source codes. Their main area of focus is universities and other research institutions as they provide a measure of researcher's productivity.
- PLOS. This tool has been available since 2009. It provides cites in recognized citation indexes and captures data from social networks and platforms where the article has been referenced or uploaded. Information on the usage of an article is also provided as a function of time.

9.3   Tips and Tricks for a Successful Submission

Despite the increasing tendency by many researchers to communicate their scholarly work through the Web, publication in peer-reviewed journals remains a vital target for those who wish to preserve high-quality standards in their professional level and secure a successful career progression. The continued dependency of researchers on publications, as expressed in the phrase "publish or perish," has resulted in an overwhelming number of submitted manuscripts to many frontline biomedical journals [9, 10]. The majority, however, of these papers are rejected for not meeting standard requirements of medical writing [11, 12]. It is therefore important that prospective authors adhere to certain methodological details in order to create a high-quality scholarly work, appropriate for publishing. So far, certain guidelines have been developed aiming to ensure transparency and completeness of reporting and enhance the credibility of research. Examples of them represent the STROBE statement [13] (designed for observational studies), the CONSORT statement [14] (aiming at improving the reporting of randomized control trials), and the PRISMA statement for reporting systematic reviews and meta-analyses [15]. As most submitted papers follow the IMRaD format [16], which established introduction, methods, results, and discussion as constituent parts of a current scientific article, we will analyze some important tips and tricks for each of these constituent sections of an article.

9.3.1 Title of the Manuscript

It is the first important element in medical writing, as it introduces the paper to the editor and reviewers and can serve as indexing label to medical libraries. Ideally, it should feature the following qualities:

- Announce the main topic of the work and attract the readers' attention.
- Be concise, accurate, complete, and specific.
- Include, if possible, key words usable for indexing and search.
- It can include the results or the answer to the review question.

9.3.2 Abstract

A properly structured abstract should summarize accurately within the limited number of words, set by the instructions for authors (usually 150–250 words), the background, materials, methodology, key findings, and final conclusion of the project. Therefore, it should be written at the conclusion of the manuscript and before its submission. It usually follows the format of the main text, featuring the following sections:

- Background or Introduction. It should be limited to a couple of sentences, exposing the problem and stating the aim of the study.
- Methods. It should include very briefly study design, setting of the study, dates of recruitment, eligibility criteria, and primary outcome of interest.
- Results. It should convey information on follow-up and dropout rates and present the key finding of the study. The reader should be convinced that the results of the study address the research question described in the background section.
- Conclusion. It should express emphatically a "take-home message" to the readership, implying either a change to or reiteration of the already followed practice.

9.3.3 Introduction

It should encompass the following topics a brief description of the problem with emphasis on its epidemiology, reference to the established methods of treatment, gap of knowledge with respect to the "gold standard" treatments that allow for the potential development of alternative treatments, purpose of the study, formulation of the study hypothesis, study type. The most critical part of the Introduction section is its last paragraph which should describe in the most clear and direct way the author's aim in preparing the submitted manuscript.

9.3.4 Materials and Methods

Probably the most important section of the manuscript as it should describe in details the included patients' population and the methodology used for the analysis.

It is advisable that this section follows the PICO format [17] (participants (eligibility, inclusion, and exclusion criteria), intervention (surgeon, surgery, rehabilitation), comparator or control (operative versus non operative, type of surgery versus other type of surgery), outcome measure). The authors should provide details on the following aspects:

- Study design. Study design, setting in which the study took place and issues of ethical approval should be addressed. Moreover, in cases of randomized control trials (RCTs), the exact method of random allocation used should be adequately presented.
- Study population. Details of baseline characteristics and demographics of the included population should be provided. Furthermore, a clear account of eligibility criteria (inclusion and exclusion criteria) should be given.
- Interventions. In case of operative intervention, not only its technical aspects should be described completely, but also the operator(s) (and level of experience in performing such a procedure) should be stated. If several surgeons were involved, details on their level of experience and expertise should be also given.
- Comparator or control group. When a new therapy is compared to an existing one, a group of individuals, serving as controls, is used. Details on the "matching process" between the treatment and control groups on various confounding variables are of paramount importance, as they are indicative of potentially existing confounding bias that would distort the validity of the study's results.
- Outcome. It is the effect of the intervention. Outcome measures used in the study should be validated. It is also important for clinical studies to include functional outcome measures (at least, one disease-specific, such as Oxford hip score, and a generic health outcome measure, such as SF-36).
- Statistics. The statistical issues that should be clearly addressed in this section are the following:
  - Power of the study and sample size. Power analysis is typically performed at the beginning of the research project and is invaluable in determining the required resources needed to perform the study and, particularly, the required sample size to determine significance when it actually occurs. Power of a study is the probability of finding a significant association when one truly exists and is defined as 1 – probability of type II error. As the probability of type II error is usually set by convention at 0.20, then the respective power of the study is 0.80, meaning that there is 80% chance that the study will detect a difference when one truly exists. The power of a study is very important as it reflects the validity of the results, particularly, when no significant association is demonstrated. Power of a study is related to sample size, meaning that when the sample size is small, the respective study might be underpowered. Readers of research reports need to know the required sample size for a clinically meaningful difference to be truly detected (with a probability above 80%). As power analysis and sample size calculations are typically performed at the beginning of a research project, respective details should appear in the methods section of the article.
  - Appropriate use of statistical tests, based on dataset distribution (parametric or nonparametric tests) and type of data (nominal, continuous, or discrete).

9.3.5 Follow-Up

Follow-up data should be complete and include the following:

- Duration of follow-up. Early clinical results usually require 1–2 years of follow-up, while midterm and long-term results would require 5 and 8–10 years of follow-up, respectively.
- Frequency of follow-up visits.
- Outcome assessor at each follow-up visit. Was he involved in the therapeutic management of the patients or was he totally blinded to the preceded treatment? These are invaluable details and give the readership an idea of potentially existing detection bias.

9.3.6 Results

This section should be brief and concise. The authors should avoid duplication of data (e.g., information presented in tables should not be repeated in the main text). This section should include the following elements:

- Recruitment. Dates defining the period of recruitment and duration of follow-up.
- Presentation of baseline characteristics and demographic data of the study population (preferably in table format).
- Details regarding participants in the study as well as losses to follow-up. Calculating loss to follow-up may be somewhat intriguing. For retrospective studies, all individuals receiving treatment during the study period should be used as the denominator, not just those with complete data. As for RCTs, the denominator for each group is the number of patients who were randomized and not those who received treatment. Loss-to-follow-up rate is very important in determining a study's validity, as usually patients lost to follow-up have different prognosis than those who completed the study. As a rule of thumb, loss to follow-up <5% leads to little bias, while >20% poses a significant threat to validity of results (attrition bias) [18, 19].
- Outcomes. For both primary and secondary outcomes presentation of the effect size along with respective confidence intervals.
- Ancillary analyses, such as subgroup analyses, adjusted analyses, etc.

9.3.7 Discussion

Writing this section is a challenging task for the authors, as they will attempt to generalize their findings. This should be done in a methodological way. For this purpose, the following steps are recommended:

- Short restatement of the main results of the study that answer the research question.
- Interpretation and general applicability of the findings of the study.

- Explanations for any conflicting or unexplained results.
- Limitations of the study and addressing potential sources of bias.
- Provide suggestions for future research directions with respect to your initial hypothesis.

9.3.8 Conclusions

This section should summarize three basic elements:

- The findings of the study, with respect to research question.
- A take-home message.
- Provide a suggestion for future direction of research on related to the topic of your work.

9.3.9 Acknowledgments

They should be listed before the reference section. They usually include funding sources as well as colleagues (other than the authors) who provided any help in the preparation or for the improvement of the manuscript.

9.4 Common Mistakes and How to Prevent Them

As a general rule, the overall quality of the manuscript in regard to proper use of grammar and syntax rules is of paramount importance. Misspelling, typing errors, and poor syntax should be avoided as they predispose negatively the reviewers and increase the likelihood of rejection. The final version of the manuscript should be thoroughly reviewed by the authors for accurate flow, syntax, and spelling.

The commonest mistakes, associated with the distinct sections of an article, are listed below.

9.4.1 Introduction

- Insufficient background information on the topic and inappropriate review of the literature.
- Lack of a clear research question statement and research objectives.

9.4.2 Methods Section

- Inappropriate study design. In RCTs, for example, a biased allocation of comparison groups is a frequent cause of selection bias.
- Inadequate handling of "dropouts," introducing attrition bias to the final results.

- Lack of power analysis. When the sample size of a research project is insufficient, the respective results cannot be considered valid and robust. Therefore, early power calculation, during the research process, is strongly advocated to determine the required sample size and appropriate resources.

9.4.3 Results

- Errors in calculating the results. The calculated rates of outcomes do not add up to 100%.
- Incorrect use of statistical tests. As most biological data are not normally distributed, the use of nonparametric tests should be preferred, unless the normality of data distribution is evident or proven. For the same reason, reporting the median and range (instead of mean and standard deviation) is preferable, when dealing with continuous data.
- Poor quality figures and tables.

9.4.4 Discussion

- Failure to discuss the significance of findings.
- Conclusions that were not substantiated by the presented results.
- Failure to discuss the limitations of the study.

9.4.5 Conclusion

- Failure to address the study question.

9.5 Take-Home Messages

- New metric tools, focusing on individual article level rather than journal level, are continuously evolving, aiming to improve the assessment of scholarly work in the modern Web-based environment.
- The art of orthopedic medical writing and publishing, vital for knowledge dissemination and career advancement, is not an easy task.
- Although an expanding volume of research material within the field of orthopedics is being produced, only a small portion of it is ultimately considered appropriate for publishing.
- Certain guidelines have been developed to ensure transparency and completeness in reporting, such as the CONSORT statement for RCTs, the STROBE statement for observational studies, and PRISMA statement for systematic reviews and meta-analyses.
- Strict adherence to certain methodological details, such as an original research question, a valid study design, a proper statistical documentation of the

results, and a well-structured manuscript written in a lucid and flowing language with appropriate syntax, are the minimal prerequisites for a successful publication.

References

1. Journal Impact factor. http://admin-pps.webofknowledge.com/JCR/help/h_impfact.htm. Accessed 25 Sept 2015.
2. San Francisco Declaration on Research Assessment. http://am.ascb.org/dora/. Accessed 25 Sept 2015.
3. Bornmann L, Williams R. How to calculate the practical significance of citation impact differences? An empirical example from evaluative institutional bibliometrics using adjusted predictions and marginal effects. J Informet. 2013;7(2):562–74. https://doi.org/10.1016/j.joi.2013.02.005.
4. Bastow S, Dunleavy P, Tinkler J. The impact of the social sciences. London: Sage; 2014.
5. Hirsch JE. An index to quantify an individual's research output. Proc Natl Acad Sci U S A. 2005;102(46):16569–72. https://doi.org/10.1073/pnas.0507655102.
6. Priem J, Taraborelli D, Groth P, Neylon C. Altmetrics: a manifesto, 26 October 2010. http://altmetrics.org/manifesto. Accessed 25 Sept 2015.
7. Piwowar H. Altmetrics: value all research products. Nature. 2013;493(7431):159.
8. Shema H, Bar-Ilan J, Thelwall M. Do blog citations correlate with a higher number of future citations? Research blogs as a potential source for alternative metrics. J Assoc Inf Sci Technol. 2014;65(5):1018–27. https://doi.org/10.1002/asi.23037.
9. Thompson DF, Callen EC, Nahata MC. New indices in scholarship assessment. Am J Pharm Educ. 2009;73:111.
10. Cole AL. Academic freedom and the publish or perish paradox in schools of education. Teach Educ Q. 2000;27:33–48.
11. Barron JP. The uniform requirements for manuscripts submitted to biomedical journals recommended by the International committee of medical journal editors. Chest. 2006;129: 1098–9.
12. International Committee of Medical Journal Editors. Uniform requirements for manuscripts submitted to biomedical journals: writing and editing for biomedical publication. 2010. http://www.icmje.org/urmfull.pdf.
13. von Elm E, Altman DG, Egger M, Pocock SJ, Gøtzsche PC, Vandenbroucke JP, STROBE Initiative. The strengthening the reporting of observational studies in epidemiology (STROBE) statement: guidelines for reporting observational studies. Int J Surg. 2014;12(12):1495–9. https://doi.org/10.1016/j.ijsu.2014.07.013.
14. Schulz KF, Altman DG, Moher D, CONSORT Group. CONSORT 2010 statement: updated guidelines for reporting parallel group randomised trials. BMC Med. 2010;8:18. https://doi.org/10.1186/1741-7015-8-18.
15. Liberati A, Altman DG, Tetzlaff J, Mulrow C, Gøtzsche PC, Ioannidis JP, Clarke M, Devereaux PJ, Kleijnen J, Moher D. The PRISMA statement for reporting systematic reviews and meta-analyses of studies that evaluate healthcare interventions: explanation and elaboration. BMJ. 2009;339:b2700. https://doi.org/10.1136/bmj.b2700.
16. Huth EJ. Structured abstracts for papers reporting clinical trials. Ann Intern Med. 1987;106(4):626–7.
17. Schardt C, Adams M, Owens T. Utilization of the PICO framework to improve searching PubMed. BMC Med Inform Decis Mak. 2007;7:16.
18. Sacket DL, Richardson WS, Rosenberg W, et al. Evidence-based medicine: how to practice and teach EBM. New York: Churchill Livingstone; 1997.
19. Bhandari M, Guyatt GH, Swiontkowski MF. User's guide to the orthopaedic literature: how to use an article about a surgical therapy. J Bone Joint Surg Am. 2001;83(6):916–26.

Open-Access Journals: The Future of Scientific Publishing?

Philip F. Stahel and Todd VanderHeiden

10.1 What is Open-Access Publishing?

The open-access publishing initiative started in the 1990s with the introduction of the World Wide Web that made the Internet available around the globe. The open-access publishing concept entails that scientific content is provided online to readers, free of charge. The "Public Library of Science" (PloS) was one of the first nonprofit open-access platforms launched with tremendous success in the early twenty-first century [1, 2]. Open-access publishing provides several unprecedented advantages compared to standard print journals [3]. This includes the timely, unrestricted, free access to scientific knowledge by any reader with access to the Internet, by eliminating financial barriers related to expensive journal subscriptions and by reducing the usual time delay of several months (or years) from the time a scientific discovery is made until the information is available to the end user.

The following apparent benefits represent intuitive incentives for authors to consider open-access publishing:

P.F. Stahel (✉)
Department of Orthopaedics, University of Colorado, School of Medicine and Denver Health Medical Center, Denver, CO, USA

Department of Neurosurgery, University of Colorado, School of Medicine and Denver Health Medical Center, Denver, CO, USA
e-mail: philip.stahel@dhha.org

T. VanderHeiden
Department of Orthopaedics, University of Colorado, School of Medicine and Denver Health Medical Center, Denver, CO, USA

© Springer International Publishing AG 2018
C. Mauffrey, M.M. Scarlat (eds.), *Medical Writing and Research Methodology for the Orthopaedic Surgeon*, https://doi.org/10.1007/978-3-319-69350-7_10

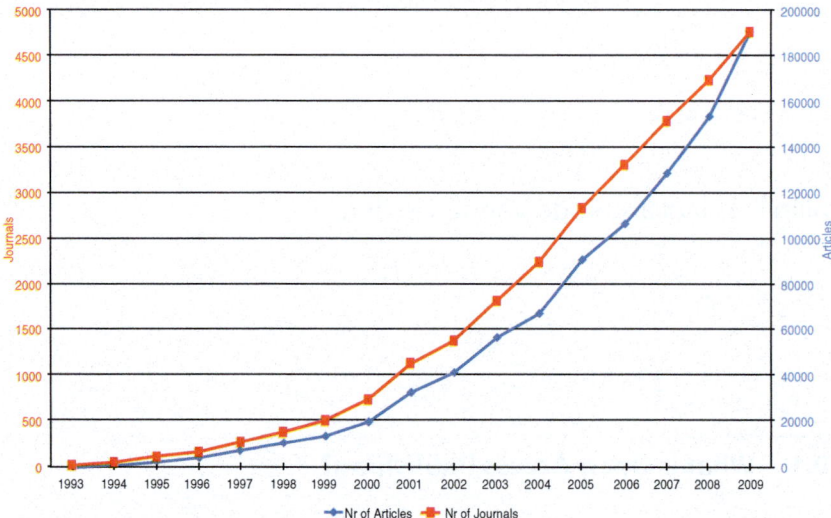

Fig. 10.1 The development of open-access publishing 1993–2009. Image adapted from [5]. Copyright 2011 Creative Commons license

- The fast-track digital publication process allows for short turnaround times of submitted manuscripts and timely publication and dissemination of the scientific work.
- All open-access articles that are published under the Creative Commons license are free to read, copy, reproduce, and distribute, as long as the original source is adequately cited.
- Authors retain the full unrestricted copyright on the entire article. This allows for replicating data and figures in future publications (e.g., review articles or book chapters) without the need for requesting a copyright release by the publisher.
- There is no limit to the length of an individual article, including the number of tables and figures.
- There are no extra charges for publishing color figures.
- All open access are archived in public repositories, including PubMed Central, in compliance with the NIH Public Access Policy [4].

The launch of new online open-access journals has seen an exponential rise from the early 1990s into the twenty-first century (Fig. 10.1) [5].

10.2 The Success Story of a New Independent Open-Access Journal

In the early stages of open-access publishing, new journals were mainly founded by independent academicians who were dissatisfied with the predominant subscription-restricted paradigm of standard print journals. We provide a brief anecdotal story from inception to publication of our own independent open-access journal that is currently celebrating its tenth anniversary. "Patient Safety in Surgery" (www.pssjournal.com) was launched in 2007 as the first and currently exclusive peer-reviewed and PubMed-cited online journal in the field of surgical patient safety [6]. The *Journal* was designed to fill an essential void by providing a forum for discussion, analysis, and work-up of system and process failures, technical complications, medical errors, and other adverse events in the management of surgical patients in the perioperative setting [6]. This scientific forum was created to lower the threshold for reporting adverse events in surgery, with the long-term goal of increasing the safety and quality of surgical care across the globe. In 2017, "Patient Safety in Surgery" remains the sole "niche" journal devoted to this important topic [7]. The conception of the journal's mission originated by a group of surgeon colleagues who brainstormed about options to improve reporting of surgical complications and adverse events in a transparent fashion [8]. We speculated about new options for sharing root causes of surgical complications, unnecessary surgery, and preventable medical errors which represent the third leading cause of death in the United States [9, 10]. These discussions led to the idea of launching a new journal to allow extrapolating this important debate to an international open platform [8]. With strong support from the publisher, BioMed Central (BMC) [11], the new journal, was successfully launched on November 7, 2007, accompanied by the first two peer-reviewed articles [12, 13]. We were astonished by the unexpected "avalanche" of submitted case reports on surgical complications and preventable sentinel events, starting within the first weeks of the journal's launch [13, 14], ongoing into the journal's tenth annual volume at present [15]. Within a short period of time of its inception, "Patient Safety in Surgery" had a spectacular beginning. The journal has been accepted and cited in PubMed from the day of its first publication. The readers' access to papers published on the journal's website (www.pssjournal.com) had increased from less than 2,000 hits in 2007 up to 16,000 accesses per month within the first few years (Fig. 10.2) [8]. Impressively, the journal is currently being read and accessed online in more than 180 countries worldwide (Fig. 10.3) [8]. These metrics support the notion of improved visibility and transparency of the new open-access publication model, even for smaller independent online journals, such as "Patient Safety in Surgery."

10.3   Shortcomings and Dangers of Open-Access Publishing

Online journals have received and unjustified poor reputation due to non-credible business enterprises that abuse the scientific mission of open-access publishing for pure pecuniary gain with a fast return on investment. Such unethical practices—termed "predatory publishing"—have received increased media coverage in recent years [16, 17].

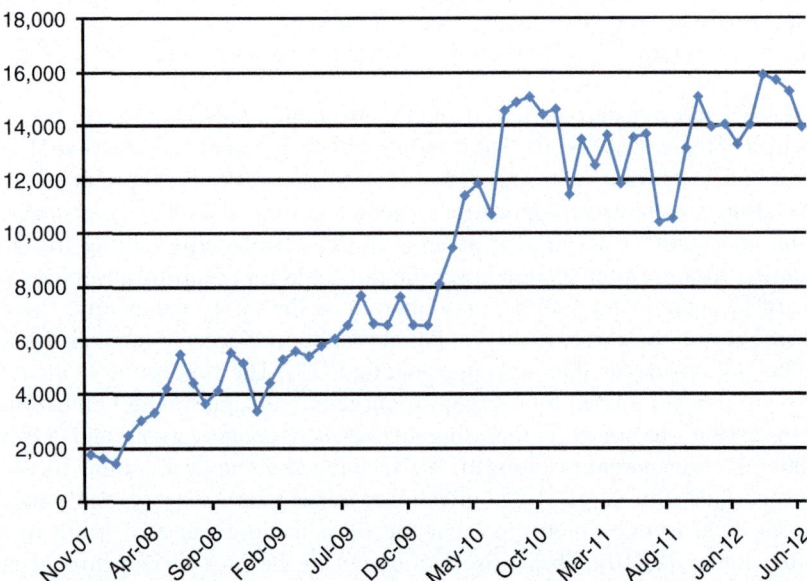

Fig. 10.2 Article downloads from the open-access journal "Patient Safety in Surgery." The graph shows the growing number of accesses to articles published from the time of the journal's launch in November 2007 until June 2012. The data reflect access statistics to the journal's website exclusively, and do not include additional sources of access, including PubMed and other portals and article repositories. Image adapted from [8]. Copyright 2012 Creative Commons license

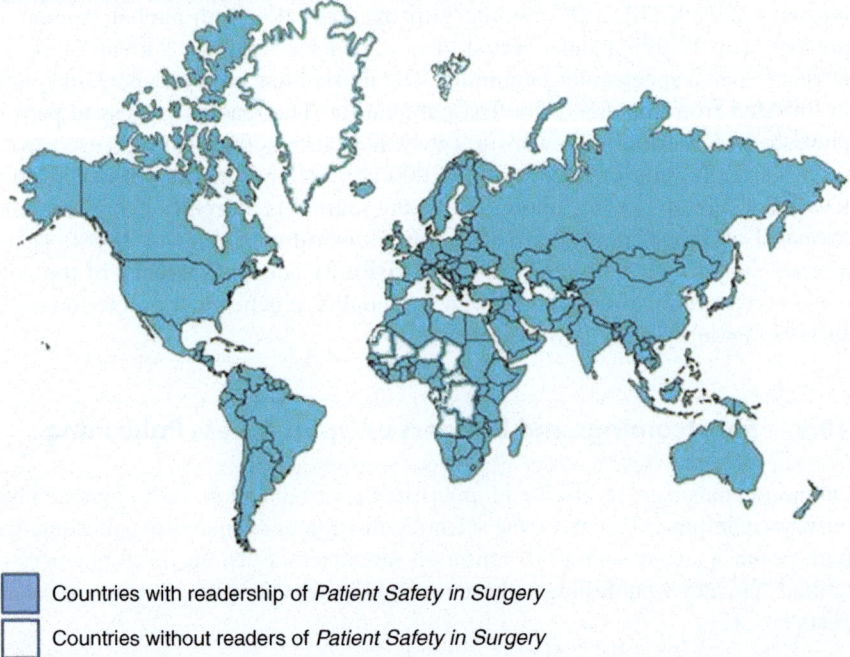

Fig. 10.3 Global readership of the open-access journal "Patient Safety in Surgery" in 2012. All countries with documented downloads of articles published in the journal are marked in blue background. Image adapted from [8]. Copyright 2012 Creative Commons license

Other worrisome reports describe a new pattern of peer-review fraud by which submitting authors falsify the contact information of solicited referees, with the goal of diverting the peer review request to their own e-mail account under a falsified name. A recent news report unveiled a fraudulent peer review scheme that led to a journal's retraction of 60 publications [18]. Since open-access journals rely on online submission and review process by default, the true prevalence of peer review fraud may be higher than currently appreciated [19]. In addition, the ever-increasing competitiveness in research under the "publish or perish!" paradigm incentivizes researchers to accept invitations from online journals of questionable scientific integrity and to split results from a single study into multiple papers, in order to increase the "n" of their scientific oeuvre in the current times of limited grant funding opportunities and increased competition [20].

10.4   Take-Home Message

Open-access publishing represents a new evolving paradigm for the timely dissemination of scientific knowledge around the globe. The intuitive advantage consists of the fast-track publication process with short times from manuscript submission until availability of the final article in the online open-access arena. In addition, authors retain the full copyright of their work which allows free dissemination and reproduction of their work through the Creative Commons license (see images reproduced in this book chapter, as a supportive example). Shortcomings of the open-access modality include the high publication fees carried by the submitting authors and the risk of fraudulent peer review and illegitimate publications of poor scientific value. In essence, authors will have to decide on the ideal target journal of choice by weighing the advantages of short publication times and global visibility of their work against the risks associated with the new publishing modality, compared to publishing in more traditional print journals.

Conflict of Interest   Both authors are editors on the editorial board of the open-access journal "Patient Safety in Surgery." The authors declare no other conflict of interest.

References

1. Bernstein P, Cohen B, MacCallum C, Parthasarathy H, Patterson M, Siegel V. PLoS Biology – we're open. PLoS Biol. 2003;1:E34.
2. Eckdahl T. Review of: PLoS Biology – a freely available, open access online journal. Cell Biol Educ. 2004;3:15–7.
3. Tennant JP, Waldner F, Jacques DC, Masuzzo P, Collister LB, Hartgerink CH. The academic, economic and societal impacts of Open Access: an evidence-based review. F1000 Res. 2016;5:632.
4. https://publicaccess.nih.gov/policy.htm. Accessed 4 Dec 2016.
5. Laakso M, Welling P, Bukvova H, Nyman L, Björk BC, Hedlund T. The development of open access journal publishing from 1993 to 2009. PLoS One. 2011;6:e20961.
6. Stahel PF, Clavien PA, Hahnloser D, Smith WR. A new journal devoted to patient safety in surgery: the time is now! Patient Saf Surg. 2007;1:1.
7. www.pssjournal.com. Accessed 4 Dec 2016.

 8. Stahel PF, Smith WR, Hahnloser D, Nigri G, Mauffrey C, Clavien PA. The 5th anniversary of 'Patient Safety in Surgery' – from the journal's origin to its future vision. Patient Saf Surg. 2012;6:24.
 9. Makary MA, Daniel M. Medical error – the third leading cause of death in the US. BMJ. 2016;353:i2139.
10. Stahel PF, VanderHeiden T, Kim F. Why do surgeons continue to perform unnecessary surgery? Patient Saf Surg. 2017. (in press).
11. www.biomedcentral.com. Accessed 4 Dec 2016.
12. Papadimos TJ, Grabarczyk JL, Grum DF, Hofmann JP, Marco AP, Khuder SA. Implementation of an antibiotic nomogram improves postoperative antibiotic utilization and safety in patients undergoing coronary artery bypass grafting. Patient Saf Surg. 2007;1:2.
13. Moore JB, Hasenboehler EA. Orchiectomy as a result of ischemic orchitis after laparoscopic inguinal hernia repair: case report of a rare complication. Patient Saf Surg. 2007;1:3.
14. Weiss HR. Adolescent Idiopathic Scoliosis – case report of a patient with clinical deterioration after surgery. Patient Saf Surg. 2007;1:7.
15. Ten Hagen A, Doldersum P, van Raaij T. Anaphylactic shock during cement implantation of a total hip arthroplasty in a patient with underlying mastocytosis: case report of a rare intraoperative complication. Patient Saf Surg. 2016;10:25.
16. Boumil MM, Salem DN. In… and out: open access publishing in scientific journals. Qual Manag Health Care. 2014;23:133–7.
17. Gasparyan AY, Nurmashev B, Voronov AA, Gerasimov AN, Koroleva AM, Kitas GD. The pressure to publish more and the scope of predatory publishing activities. J Korean Med Sci. 2016;31:1874–8.
18. Fountain H. Science journal pulls 60 papers in peer-review fraud. The New York Times, July 11, 2014.
19. Stahel PF, Moore EE. Peer review for biomedical publications: we can improve the system. BMC Med. 2014;12:179.
20. Stahel PF, Clavien PA, Smith WR, Moore EE. Redundant publications in surgery: a threat to patient safety? Patient Saf Surg. 2008;2:6.

The manufacturer's authorised representative in the EU is Springer
Nature Customer Service Centre GmbH, Europaplatz 3, 69115 Heidelberg,
Germany. If you have any concerns regarding our products, please
contact ProductSafety@springernature.com

Printed and bound by CPI Group (UK) Ltd, Croydon, CR0 4YY
23/04/2026
02095586-0006